Preface

Learn mind-body techniques to raise your vibrations and achieve your potential through personal transformation, awakenings of all kinds including synchronicity and ultimately a persistent enlightenment.

Learn techniques to excel in every way with effective sound therapy and brainwave entrainment, including advanced learning, relaxation, meditation, rejuvenation, pranayama, and awakenings of the mind. Enjoy life more with this amazing journey and greater personal power.

Become more successful and healthier than ever by getting a better handle on stress. Learn effective mind-body techniques for relaxation and rejuvenation, to rebound and heal quickly while learning to become more resilient to stress and its impact on the immune system.

Learn to enjoy life more with this incredible journey, greater personal power, clarity of mind, inner peace, love and joy, as your life flows with synchronicity, with greater intuition and awareness, you effortlessly manifest your personal desires reflected in your external life. This is a great place to be and what should be a major layover on any path to enlightenment, while exploring and gaining experience.

Take it Step by Step! This book will help you take everything to the next level while progressively increasing health, wellbeing, awakenings, synchronicity, and even the opportunity to experience the ultimate reality for yourself, in a highly vibrant and joyful way!

Stress Relief That Works! Apply these techniques for prevention and wellbeing, and help with chronic conditions and diseases, including pain, depression, anxiety, and fatigue, and even accelerate healing in a very organic and stress free kind of way, by simply restoring and improving your state of mind and immune response, which often suffers from all the modern day stressors of life.

Restore Your Youth! Allow your mind body to perform as well, if not better, than it once did in your youth, from energy and stamina to healing, it's all much easier than you might expect. Discover how to energize your life effectively with a greater understanding of those things that are influencing your energy levels.

Raise your vibrations to new heights to expand your consciousness, creativity, intuition, innovation, awareness, and amazingly become healthier, more energetic, and increase your attraction in a very synchronicity sort of way!

Get this book in Paperback, Kindle Edition, or Kindle Download App Edition while promotional prices last. Energizing your life and wellbeing can start today!

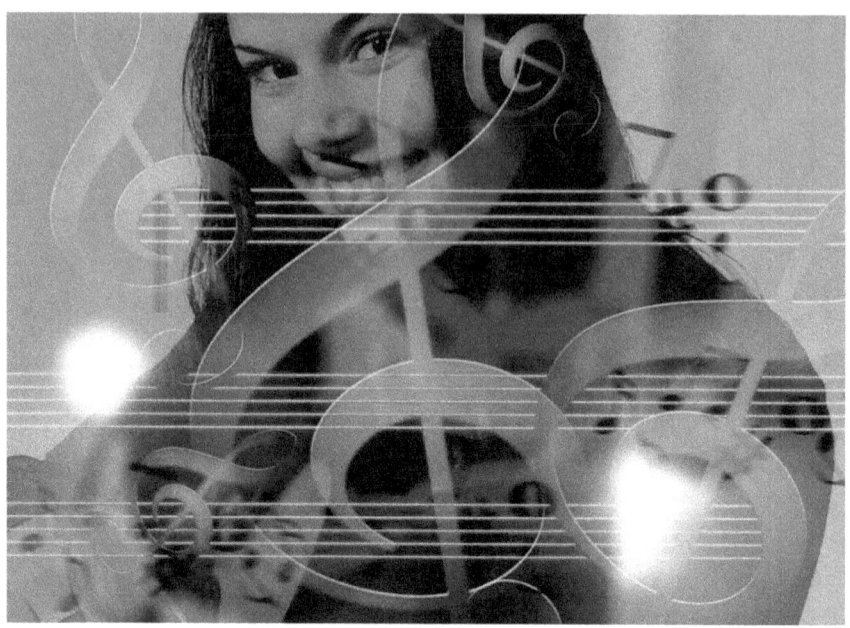

About the Author

Dan Harp is a mind-body expert who has experienced many awakenings on all levels, ultimately achieving enlightenment. Now for the first time, he is sharing his firsthand knowledge and experience to help you find the way, rise above your challenges and enjoy a truly healthy, energized and enlightened lifestyle. His books often venture well beyond similar books, with in-depth coverage, plenty of real world explanations and how-to guidance.

If you like the book, please take a moment to do a review of Healthy Vibrations at: http://www.amazon.com/dp/1530003458

As a Thank You for your interest in Dan Harp's books, he has a special gift for you, one of his latest releases.

Free eBook Give Away for You

Top 50 Best "Stress Busting" Smoothies

Stress Management Made Easy

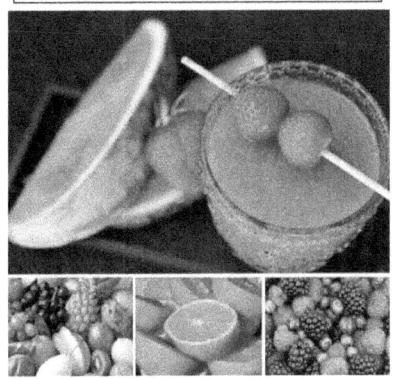

You will find the secret URL and Coupon at the back of this book

Healthy Vibrations Contact Information:
AbundantEnergyDesires@gmail.com?subject=Healthy%20Vibrations%20Inquiry

Ordering Information:

Quantity sales - Special discounts are available on quantity purchases by corporations, associations, academics, and others. For details, contact the publisher at the email address above.

This book is available at Amazon in Paperback, the Kindle, and the Amazon Any Device App Editions.

Books by Dan Harp, including paperback editions, can be found at Author Central.

Author Central
http://www.amazon.com/author/danharp

Table of Contents

Chapter II – The Metaphysical Experience   73

Chapter I – The Physical Energy Influences

Shakti and Prana Energy Influences as Life-Giving Forces

Cosmic Energy is the Hindu translation of "Shakti" which means "Empowerment" or "Power" and represents the dynamic forces thought to move through the entire universe. Shakti is the personification of the divine feminine power responsible for creation and the agent of change.

The various cultural terms includes Hindu Shakti, Prana, Apana and Yyana, Chinese Chi (Qi), Polynesian Mana, Vietnamese Khi, Korean Gi, Japanese Ki, subtle energy and woo energy, Hebrew koach-ha-guf, Greek Bios, English Aether, Cosmic Energy, Kundalini Energy, Natural Energy, and Material Energy, American Indians Orenda, Ancient Germans Od, and Scientifically known as Dark Matter, most of which are believed to be a part of any living thing, translating to breath, air, gas, or life force that permeates the universe.

In essence, anything that is alive has Shakti for energy, vibrant health, strong emotions, feeling good, feeling life has meaning and value, energy to engage life for growth and fulfillment, and to expand your consciousness.

In short, Shakti is the fuel that powers your spiritual growth and awakenings.

In physics, there are four distinct states of matter that are solid, liquid, gas and plasma. Although Shakti plasma may exist, it would be in space, not here on Earth.

Prana is simply Shakti Air. Although you can only fill your lungs with air, you can fill your entire subtle body (the space your body occupies) with Shakti Air.

Pranayama is the practice of a specific and intricate breathing technique in yoga and refers to various techniques for accumulating expanding, and working with prana.

Some of the best "enhanced" breathing techniques include:

- Breath in prana to each of your chakras.

- Breath in prana to your entire body.

- Breathe from different parts of your body to bring Shakti vapors to your lungs from different parts of your body.

- Exhale quickly if you have some form of Shakti powder or vapors that you don't like, especially if it tastes more chemical than living Shakti flora, or especially if it is too overpowering and feels like a bad drug. This will help to train your body to "smoke" the Shakti rather than "burn" it into vapors.

- Separate the prana in your mouth using your tongue, and then push it up to your brain.

- All of this takes practice, which can be easier when you have some Shakti you would like to expel.

- Once you have mastered breathing, the next way to expel something you don't want is to simply focus on it and let it flow free on your exhale or guide it through your body. This is also a great way to meet women, by putting it in their aura, especially something with a floral scent, assuming they are awake enough to sense it on some level.

Shakti has its own periodic table, supporting life, molecules of all kinds, and has its own energy density. The only difference is how it is perceived and some of its properties are somewhat different. Here are the more significant Shakti physics properties:

- Exists in at least Solid, Liquid and Gaseous states.

- Strong Force exists, electromagnetic forces can be sensed by the body, but they are not the same as ordinary matter, and not detectable by current technology.

- Prana is the Shakti equivalent of air, where you can fill your lungs with ordinary air and direct Shakti air (prana) to anywhere in the body. This along with many examples of composite Shakti would suggest a periodic table similar to ordinary matter, perhaps in the same order.

- Shakti can occupy and pass through other Skakti and Ordinary Matter with resistance relative to the frequencies involved.

- The size of any mass is relative to the observer. Consciously, Shakti can be compressed when drawn in and consumed. The smaller you make it, the denser the molecules become, which makes taste and smell more pungent.

- Shakti can be burned in the body into a vapor for the brain. The breakdown of Shakti may ultimately be a cold fission process. Normally, Shakti will get larger and less dense as it breaks down, and the taste and smell is diluted. When fission occurs, it is a cool feeling in the body, with a lot of possibilities depending on decay method, including protons, pions, muons, photons, neutrinos and ions.

- Folding of space is common in the realm of Shakti. If you connected one end of a Shakti rope to one person and the other end to another, as these people moved away from each other, the Skakti will go more out-of-phase, but once they are in proximity again, it returns to its original phase.

- Some Shakti, especially subtle body parts, are strongly interactive, all of which suggests there could be more than one type of Shakti.

- Entirely similar to a 5th dimension, but exists in our space-time. This could probably be described better as we live in a reality of dualities on so many levels, including matter-energy, particles-waves, matter-vibrations, energy-frequencies, ordinary matter-Shakti, etc.

Signs of positive Shakti awareness include:

- Your eyes are clear and bright

- You have the power to take a full breath

- You feel vitality and full of energy

- You have a clear mind

- You have a good memory

- You have the ability to deeply relax

- You have the ability to fall asleep and get a good night's rest

- You face the stress with resilience and courage

- You have both an inner and outer glow

- You can easily digest life experiences

- You have the ability to expel toxins from your subtle body and mind

- You have fewer than usual emotions

- People are drawn to you more than usual

- You may experience some Shakti that vaporizes in a manic, superman, drug, or even bad drug sort of way, so this is where it is good to know the breathing techniques.

Indian philosophy states that Shakti creative power has three states. These three Shakti's can be thought of as intention, formulation and expression. For example, you intend to do something, you formulate a plan in your mind, and you act on that plan, expressing your inner state into the outer world. You create something.

- ***Gyana (jnana) Shakti*** – the power to know

- ***Iccha Shakti*** – willpower

- ***Kriya Shakti*** – the power to act

Yoga philosophy describes three forms of Shakti moving through the body, mind and spirit:

- ***Prana Shakti*** governs all organs and physical actions. Cultivate this form of Shakti via deep relaxation techniques such as Yoga Nidra and with Pranayama.

- ***Chitta Shakti*** governs all of your mental functions, including your intelligence, thinking, emotions, memory, desires, courage, decision making, planning and so on.

- **Atma Shakti** is the causal and creative power of consciousness. Develop spiritual Shakti by techniques such as those found using Chakras.

There is a simpler way to relate to Shakti from personal experience:

- **Prana Shakti** – Shakti Air

- **Active Shakti** – Includes Shakti produced by the subtle body for emotions and intellectual endeavors, which enters the body at the base of the tongue and doesn't need to be vaporized to be somewhat available. Also includes some Shakti's in liquid forms.

- **Passive Shakti** – Includes Shakti generally in the form of solids that needs to be vaporized in order to sense.

This guide is intended to raise your awareness and understanding regarding your subtle body, how to manage it, the pitfalls to watch out for, and how to be more selective about the Shakta flora you are using, along with guiding your through awakenings of all kind on the road to enlightenment.

Using Your Chakras with Shakti and Prana

In yogic tradition, kundalini is a primal energy based on Shakti, described as "coiled" at the base of the spine. The awakening involves moving this ancient vital energy up from the "root chakra" to the "crown chakra" at the top of the head, usually through meditation, breathing, or chanting of mantras.

The chakra system in some Indian traditions is thought to consist of energy centers in your subtle body. According to these beliefs and various esoteric and mystical teachings, the subtle body is separate from the physical body, which corresponds to a subtle plain of existence, in a greater chain of being, that culminates in the physical form. This separation of the subtle body is common amongst many cultures, which translates to things like "the most sacred body", "the light body", "the rainbow body", and "the body of bliss" and the list goes on, but we will be sticking with the term "Subtle body" throughout.

It is said to be many chakras in the subtle body, but only seven are considered important. There are many interpretations of how the chakra's work, but they all basically entail the circulation of life-energy.

Achieving ascension of the kundalini through the chakra system leads to different levels of awakening and mystical experience, until ultimately reaching spiritual awakening. This can be somewhat of a spontaneous and a figurative process involving kundalini energy from Shakti, igniting both chakras and lining.

So what is a Chakra?

You are going to laugh because there is so much misconception about these. Your subtle body has linings around it. You can pull down more linings from your crown chakra. Each chakra, from the root to the crown, is a small "coil" on this lining that bunches the lining, and is used as a focal point to ignite and extinguish Shakti.

The lining is incredibly strong and stretchable material, which could thought of as countless smaller chakras. The thickness of the lining varies too. You can pull down more linings from your crown chakra, with different Shakti ignited on each layer. So when it is said there are many chakras, the lining is made of the same material as the chakras and can be ignited directly. Once the lining is ignited, it can result in a temperature decrease of up to a couple degrees, depending on the Shakti involved and the thickness of the linings.

You don't actually need your kundalini to ignite chakras. To get something started, simply taste some Shakti and reach up to your crown chakra by extending your tongue... Well you see, your mouth, lips, tongue and eyes are amongst the few components in your body that exists in the physical world and the Shakti world, so with practice, you can extended your Shakti tongue to your crown chakra or anywhere else in your body. Furthermore, you can extend it outside your body, practically any size, which is a great way to grab Shakti floating around or even on the outside of somebody. This can also be achieved by sucking in Shakti, again where size doesn't really matter. These skills can take years of practice, so the main thing is to understand that it can be done.

Although you may find deeper understandings by manually playing with chakra's, including starting with the root chakra and working your way up, in general practice, your kundalini is an automated process that you have some control over, while your chakras can be ignited manually. To turn off chakras, simply suck on them by extending your lips over them. Your kundalini can be temporarily shut down by sucking on your root chakra.

Once you have done all the playing you want, and get good at turning chakra's on and off, it's time to raise your kundalini if it hasn't spontaneously ignited already.

A synchronicity awakening is a great place to be for a while especially if you are young. Some will want to jump right into a spiritual awakening. Eventually, you will need to decide what to do about your higher chakra.

Just so you know, your throat chakra is under your tongue, the third-eye chakra is between your eyes and the crown chakra is straight up from the center of your tongue, on the inside of your subtle body lining, like all chakras.

So what are the Differences between Chakras and a Kundalini?

Your root chakra is a coil directly over your anal canal. This is the one you want to ultimately start, either by tasting, smelling or in some way sensing the Shakti you want to use, then essentially moving it with your mind to this chakra or even licking the chakra. Start with prana, do some breathing exercises, taking prana all the way down to the chakra. This chakra can also start spontaneously from being exposed to Shakti in the environment around you, perhaps from other people.

In any case, once this chakra is ignited, your kundalini is free to start. You can use meditation to do this too, just focus on your root chakra and kundalini.

What can take years to do for some people the first time ultimately becomes so easy that you will be able to ignite any part of your lining with little to no thought at all.

Another way to go is to focus on third-eye activation which may involve detoxification and decalcification. You may find that your kundalini ignites spontaneously on its own once your third-eye is active. Once the demand for cosmic energy (Shakti vapors) increases in the brain, the body will accommodate, and raise your kundalini; which is actually a tornado like force originating from your root chakra that will stir your subtle body, making cosmic energy much more abundant and available to the brain and endocrine system. This is actually the way I did it, with a spontaneous kundalini raising.

The kundalini itself is actually a pin at the top of your anal canal. This pin carries an electric charge, and is needed to maintain proper subtle body pressure and the tornado like effect. Kundalini syndrome is an over-active kundalini that is easy to diagnosis. This can happen when the pin gets dislodged, either deliberately by someone messing with you, probably from anal sex, and perhaps other causes. In any case, the pin can be fixed by sucking upward.

Some people know how to activate an deactivate your kundalini with their minds, which can take the wind out of your sails or even activate your subtle body in a way that promotes theft of Shakti, so once you have achieved your spiritual awakening, you might want to consider learning how to do this yourself too. It's good to know. Although it's not recommended for any particular situation, you can give up the convenience of your kundalini for better control too.

For the first four years of my journey, I strictly relied on my kundalini and didn't think chakras even existed. With your subtle body, there is always more than one way to accomplish anything, but its best to keep it simple until you are ready for more advanced things.

There is extensive coverage of these topics in upcoming chapters.

Primal Energy Influences as Life-Giving Forces

Ordinary hydrogen (protons) is by far the most common atom in the universe and makes up more than 90 percent of all the atoms. Under normal temperatures and pressures is has a negative electron. Hydrogen primarily exists in a diatomic gaseous state as molecular hydrogen, which is known to have numerous therapeutic benefits.

Drinking water and eating carbohydrates gets you part of the way there, although hydrogen absorption is limited to metabolic reactions in the body yielding a neutral charge, whereas pure hydrogen in the atmosphere and environment results in even greater energy.

Several hundred scientific articles demonstrate diatomic (molecular) hydrogen to have therapeutic potential in every organ of the body and against hundreds of diseases, including the reduction of oxidative stress and oxygen radicals, upregulation of antioxidant enzymes, anti-inflammatory effects, anti-apoptotic benefits, anti-obesity effects, and anti-allergy benefits.

Therefore, anyone who needs oxygen in particular should have it accompanied with hydrogen gas, which is now considered an emerging medical gas, and in gas form is by far the most effective delivery system.

The average hydrogen content in the air at ground level is .6 parts per million, which varies and the testing methods sound like they need review. The irony here is the most abundant atom in the universe is in scarce supply when it comes to fully supporting overall health and longevity on planet earth.

Other ways to get molecular hydrogen includes a water generator that ionizes drinking water (marginal benefits), taking a bath in water rich in molecular hydrogen (device), or increasing the production of certain intestinal bacterial.

Similar effects can be observed with an ionizer device in the room, similar to the Wein VI-2500 design (450 trillion ions/sec), because many of these devices on the market today have questionable functionality and concentrations. These are also being considered in hospitals to neutralize viruses in the air and cause them to fall to the floor.

Negative ions have several hundred scientific articles to support their benefit. They are often found naturally near running water, like a stream and after a storm, or while taking a shower.

The body is capable of running hot for extended periods of time, but it comes at a price. Striving for balance, with the ability to run hot (positive energies) and/or cold (negative energies) as needed is ideal, which is often a challenge with all the stressors of modern society, at times of illness, and with the elderly in particular, considering current atmospheric and environmental conditions.

What are less understood by science are Cosmic Energy, "Shakti" and "Prana", which can be drawn from the surrounding environment with proper breathing techniques.

Pranayama is the practice of a specific and intricate breathing technique in yoga and refers to several techniques for accumulating, expanding, and working with prana in various disciplines.

Cosmic energy is actually the vapor, or gaseous, state of Shakti. Other interpretations of cosmic energy include Reiki and Therapeutic Touch.

At least one scientific theory supports the idea that Composite Shakti "transparent matter" atoms breakdown in the body to molecular hydrogen, so learning proper breathing techniques could be more effective than buying molecular hydrogen gas or devices to produce molecular hydrogen from water.

According to Dr. Patrick Flanagan, hydrogen may be the missing link to slowing down the aging process.

Environment can be an Energy Vampire

Toxic Energy Influences

The liver detoxifies substances from the bloodstream, including ammonia. It metabolizes nutrients, and regulates the amount of sugar (glucose), protein, fat and hormones that enter the bloodstream, helping your body by providing it with energy and fighting off infections.

Over time thousands of the pours in your liver become clogged. What happens is parasites die, get lodged in the pours of the liver, and then additional matter builds up around these parasites, eventually completely blocking the pours. This will significantly degrade liver performance, energy and wellbeing and results in symptoms of toxic overload.

Doing a liver cleanse is by far the best way to improve liver function. You can just search the internet for "Gallbladder and Liver Cleanse Recipe".

Gallbladder and Liver Cleanse Recipe
https://www.google.com/search?q=Gallbladder+and+Liver+Cleanse+Recipe

There are many to choose from, but they all follow the same basic approach and timing, involving drinking a lemon or grapefruit juice and drinking olive oil.

I've been doing these kinds of cleanses every couple few years for over the last 20 years now; It's an absolute must for anybody interested in rejuvenation, reversing disease or fighting cancer.

Not only will it allow you to tolerate higher treatment levels, it will help prevent cancer from metastasizing to the liver. Here are two that I've tried:

Natural Life Energy
http://www.naturallifeenergy.com/liver-gallbladder-cleanse/

Natural Liver & Gall Bladder Cleanse
http://wellnessmama.com/category/remedies/

Other foods that would help improve liver function include apples rich in pectin, avocados rich in glutathione, green tea rich in catechins, leafy green vegetables rich in chlorophylls, and cabbage, garlic and cruciferous vegetables for their enzyme benefits.

Years ago, I created a homemade juice that you need a shot glass for. It consisted of a few cloves of garlic straight up. Garlic is an incredibly hearty plant, with an enzyme based immune response. Cooking garlic kills the enzymes, but in its raw form these cloves are extremely potent, especially when they hit the blood stream all at once.

It would take a lot more than a dare to get me to do this again. You get the bed spins in no time. If nothing else, you will get an appreciating of how effective and potent enzymes can be to cleans your body.

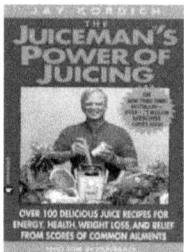 The Juiceman, Jay Kordich turned me on to homemade juices over 30 years ago. His recipes are a must try even today, He has several interesting recipes for detoxing ("Cucumber Green Tea Detox" and the "All Star Oranges, Carrots, and Apricots Detox"), cleansing ("Cranberries and Pairs") and energy ("Apple and Grape Metabolic Boost", "Orange and Mango Vitamin Boost" and the "Pair, Apple Mineral Boost"), and may more recipes to choose from.

Check out the Juiceman's website for further recipes:
http://www.juiceman.com/Recipes.aspx

Dr. Ace has an interesting 6 Step Liver Cleans that involves removing toxic foods from your diet, drinking raw vegetable juice, loading up on potassium rich foods (Tomato Sause's, Beet Greens, Spanish, Beans, Blackstrap Molasses and Bananas), Coffee Enemas, Milk Thistle, Dandelion and Turmeric Supplements, and eat real liver or take liver tablets.

Dr. Ace also has an interesting, "Secret Detox Drink" to boost energy and help you detox, with a recipe that calls for apple cider, vinegar, lemon juice, cayenne pepper, cinnamon and water.

Check out Dr. Ace's website for further details.
http://draxe.com/liver-cleanse/

These days there are numerous premade detoxification kits on the market too. Over the years I've had good luck with homeopathic treatments and supplements, but I haven't tried any of these, so I really can't vouch for them, but you can inquire at your local health store.

Parasites and Toxins are Energy Vampires.

Essential Energy Influences

There can be several causes to that feeling of "nothingness" or "emptiness", but start with shoring up your energies.

Any physical exercise can elevate brain function, mood, can be very uplifting, and even help with energy levels too. Sometimes, that's not enough though, it's more about getting the right kind of energy flowing again, or you may need to shore up your state of mind.

Routine Exercise, Diet and Sleep Goes Along Way

Even just a little exercise each day can go a long way for overall health and vitality.

Don't skip meals like breakfast, the most important meal of the day! This could just elevate stress hormone levels and drop sugar levels, which will set you back.

The other thing you shouldn't do is just one big meal a day, or skipping meals on a regular basis, because you will just be training your body to store calories, which is often going to lead to weight gain. Even a small portion of fruit and nuts is better than nothing.

The ying and yang of diet and exercise is to achieve balance, with some swings one way or other, but routine is key, especially on the intake. Some say even five smaller portions a day is better than three moderate portions a day, to get your body out of the habit of storing calories.

There is some trial and error involved to find what is right for you, but there are all kinds of resources available to research diet and exercise too.

There are various forms of yoga that can be excellent, including Karma yoga, Dhyana yoga, Ashtanga yoga, Bhakti yoga, Vinyasa yoga, and much more

Tie Chi is another practice that goes along way without impact to the joints.

In any case, exercise and diet both work best in moderation and on a semi-regular routine.

The same goes for sleeping, going to bed about the same time every night can help regulate everything and help you to feel great in the morning.

Personally, I'm more of a night owl, which isn't as cool as it sounds as you start getting older.

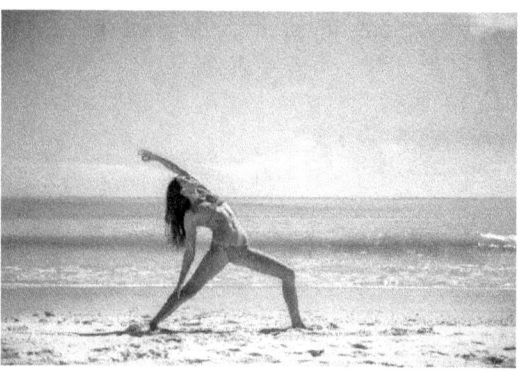

Get Your Energy Flowing Properly

Often it's just a matter of lacking the right kind of energy to rebound from feeling empty or drained. Sleep can help in some situations. Reiki may help too.

Things like yoga and meditation may help too.

The idea is to get your energy flowing properly again.

Try some breathing exercises; start with slow deep breaths in through the nose, exhale a little faster through the mouth. Now do the same thing while focusing on each of your chakras, as if breathing in from them, repeated several times. If you find resistance in the neck in particular, that's where you need to focus further sessions, and you may need to breathe in very hard from the neck to at least become more aware of the blockage and eventually clear it.

There is a lot of information online about pranayama along with prana or Shakti, which can sometimes solidify in the body.

It's best to stay active, but once you find yourself in this situation, take it to heart, because just a little exercise every day can go along way for good energy flow!

Consider a Life Coach

A life coach can help to shore up your esteem issues and figure out what you really want out of life. It might be good to find someone local, but in the meantime, here is someone who is really in the now. She goes by Kidest OM, and she can help you to live in the moment and get out of this funk; she is very inspirational.

https://www.youtube.com/results?search_query=Kidest+OM

Shore up Your Self-Esteem Issues

Overcome that anxious and nervous feeling from doing something new for the first time, which diminishes with experience.

Top 10 Activities to Overcome Self-Esteem Problems:

1. Fake it until you feel it, or should I say act the part, knowing that any situation is a performance, so your body language comes across the way you want
2. Get prepared and speak assertively, at a normal pace, without hesitations
3. Work on thinking and acting positively, focus on solutions, not negative thoughts
4. Dress the part and groom yourself for the part
5. Get to know yourself better
6. Create a mental picture of the self-image that you desire
7. Set some small goals and achieve them to get some wins under your belt
8. Volunteer for a good cause to gain experience
9. Do something you have been procrastinating about or really do any activities, even if you make mistakes, or even if they are just small things, just for the experience
10. Clean up your room or desk, this can often be an expression of your state of mind.

You can start with youtube for online courses.
https://www.youtube.com/results?search_query=self-confidence+building+exercise

Quora has some excellent answers too:
https://www.quora.com/What-are-some-life-changing-hacks

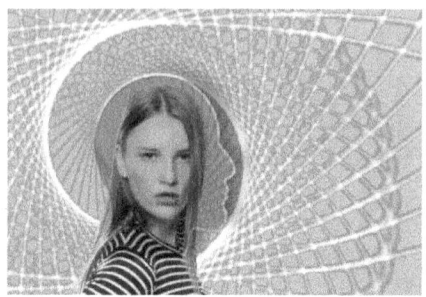

Top Reasons Why People Aren't More Successful

1. **Never step up to the plate** - Success is a participation sport
2. **Low self-esteem, self-imposed limitations and limiting beliefs** - Success has no boundaries
3. **Procrastination or apathetic** - Take a lesson from ready-fire-aim or agile mythology, lukewarm on issues doesn't pay
4. **Can't face adversary or confrontation** - Success welcomes challenges
5. **Don't understand the value of time** - Time is money
6. **Lofty goals, unrealistic goals, or poor execution** - Continuously align your goals and actions keeps you on top
7. **Under funding** - Plan for startup and growth with realistic expectations
8. **Skill gaps or complacency** - Make sure your skills align with your current and future needs. Learn on the job whenever possible
9. **Lacks discipline or focus** - Juggling competing demands for your time can be as much an art as a science.
10. **Just can't say no** - Some people will say yes just to be viewed as the good guy

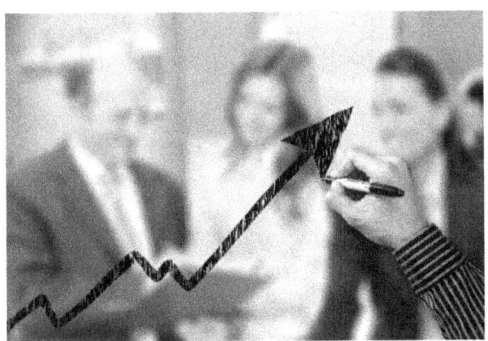

Becoming Smarter by the Day

1. **Quotes of the Day** - delivered to your inbox from famous people who have faced the same life challenges as you. This can be very insightful, inspirational and lead to wisdom.
2. **Problem Solving** - keep yourself challenged with problems to sharpen your skill sets. Become a better listener to understand problems form the perspective of others. Look at problems from every perspective possible. Make decisions.
3. **Creativity** - includes anything from creative writing, arts, crafts, videos, music, illustrations, design, coding, architecture, etc. Practice can help you go beyond analytical intelligence to create novel, interesting and unique ideas.
4. **Curiosity** - questioning everything with insatiable curiosity, and a certain amount of skepticism, rather than just accepting the status quo, will help form depth of knowledge, evaluate ideas and strengthen your neuroconnections.
5. **Self-Reflection -** meditation and brain storming can be excellent exercises to help form solutions and optimize your neuroconnections.
6. **Quora Questions** - answering questions can help you articulate your thoughts, interpret feedback and respond to replies in a way that can help you form clarity.
7. **Continued Education** - Read some non-fiction books and articles to help build your mental knowledge base. Overcome complacency and stay current in your field(s) of interest pays in the long run, with Ted Talk, YouTube, documentaries, interviews, podcasts, on-line courses, seminars and just hanging out with peers.
8. **Relaxation** - Allow yourself to rejuvenate with a good nights rest, and use music or meditation to help you relax. Learn simple techniques to overcome stress and find that optimal zen state for learning and retention.

9. **Time Management** - Learn good time management and planning skills and reduce unnecessary distractions and clutter in your life. Work and study smarter, not harder.
10. **Health** - Learn the best techniques and balance of diet and exercise to maintain peak mental and physical performance, and stay as resilient as possible to health problems of any kind.

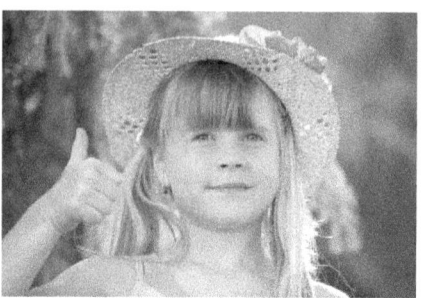

Dealing With Procrastination

Everyone struggles with doing things at times when they aren't interested in them, that are boring, that are mundane, when they have something better to do, or with things they simply don't want to do.

Procrastinators take this to new heights... Why do today what you can put off until tomorrow... This can be from overwhelming activities, things they dread, or just plain old mood or laziness.

Here are some hacks that might help:

1. Set a deadline for yourself to help make the work more challenging.
2. Work for 15 minutes just to make some progress without it being intimidating, take a 5 minute break if you want, then get back to it for another 15 minutes.
3. Break the task down into smaller chunks so it isn't so intimidating.
4. Work for 30 minutes at a time, then work on something you want for 10 minutes, and repeat until the day is done or work is complete. Give yourself a sweet reward once the work is done.
5. Focus on the possibilities and opportunities in regards to the project rather than the difficulties and obstacles.
6. Do a 5 minute burst of highly focused work to get out of procrastination mode and then decide how you want to proceed.

7. Put your phone on airplane mode and unplug, write down any nagging reminders on your mind, eliminate any other distractions, while you plan your workload and start feeling focused on the tasks at hand.
8. Set your Facebook friends to acquaintances to just get the important updates.
9. Occasionally, work from the coffee shop, backyard, or library to help improve creativity and focus on work away from the office.
10. Listen to some ambient music, brainwave entertainment or white noise to improve focus.
11. Get some houseplants to help improve creativity, focus, concentration and well-being, which is a small price to pay to have to water them.
12. Learn to say no more on tasks that just aren't right for you. Be picky about the work that you accept.
13. Delegate worthwhile tasks to your team. If it's not important enough to do that, prune your to-do-list.
14. Try some speech dictation software to get your thoughts down faster, record idea's and emails on the go.
15. Accomplish at least one important task each day and keep the trend going.
16. Eat some chocolate for a rush of dopamine that boosts motivation.
17. Reward by letting yourself be happy so you will be more likely to stay in the zone and be more productive. Take breaks to joke around, watch a funny video, and chat with a friend.
18. Finish your day with a new to-do-list that will help you get in the mindset for the following morning.
19. When you start your day, ask yourself if I could get one thing done today, what would it be? Adjust your to-do-list accordingly.
20. Spend the first hour each morning working on high priority tasks before you check your email.

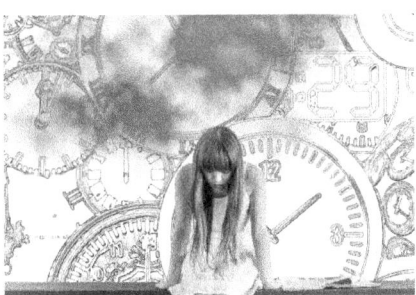

Negative Thoughts can be Energy Vampires

Emotional Energy Influences

Have you ever had someone enter a room and notice it became charged with a fresh, new energy that changes the dynamics of the entire room? People with a high energy, high vibrational frequency, often do just that, so others often enjoy having their presence around.

You can generally tell negative people by their pessimism, defeatism, cynicism, emotionalism, dramatism, and negativism. Their very attitude and feelings often gets the best of them, bringing their vibrational frequencies down with them.

These people often have a low self-esteem and vibrational frequencies that can bring others down too.

You can pick your friends, but you can't pick your family. The easiest thing to do is take these negative people in small doses. To put things in perspective, anyone who causes you stress, tension or exposes you to low vibrations could be considered a drain on you, so you need to change the dynamics of the relationship to bring them up, rather than letting them bring you down.,

Although some of these people may thrive on negative energy, including negative emotions; this is often a sign of immature development, not malice or contempt against you. They could really use the tools throughout this guide, along with a good life coach and perhaps even a good therapist, so get them a copy of this guide as a gift if you want to help. A good friend can go much further too, especially if you could show them how happiness, joy, passion and love can easy trump all, and are amongst the highest and most vibrant of all the emotions.

If you are a high energy individual, with a little work on your part, using the tools and techniques in this guide, most people won't be able to bring you down. Once you have abundant sustainable energy, while taking care of yourself in all ways, shining brightly like the stars, this kind of darkness will recede into the night.

Here is some additional food for thought when dealing with people:

- Take negative people in small doses until you become more tolerant energetically for longer periods of time, while remaining grounded to yourself.

- Trust your instincts in people, help where you can, but don't leave yourself vulnerable to anyone who instigates and thrives on negative energy and emotions from others.
- Take a deep breath, hold it, and exhale slowly while keeping your chest out and repeat, anytime you feel a drain. This is the your first best defense against any kind of Energy Vampire, incidental or intentional; including any stress or tension you may be feeling in the movement.
- Raise your shields anytime you feel a drain. As you will learn in the coming chapters, energy can be directed, re-directed and even blocked at will, merely by using your focus.
- Just say NO while you set boundaries and emotional distance until you grow thicker skin against negative people. For single encounters, getting defensive will only add to the negative charge, instead just tell them what you can do for them to resolve the issue.
- Pay attention to the type of people in your life that are negatively impacting you to see if you can discover something about yourself that you need to work on that will help you attract more vibrant people to your life. See the law of attraction under "Power Tools for Your Tool Belt".
- Spend more time with high energy friends or just getting out and having fun on your own can work wonders. Give yourself the time and space to reflect on how you feel without negative influences.

Negative Emotions can be Energy Vampires

Natural Energy Influences

Boosting Your Immune System

All you need to do is learn to relax, which is the polar opposite of stress. Your immune system is optimal in a relaxed state. Stress suppresses many immune responses, short of blood clotting, to support the release of energy needed for fight or flight, which is designed as a short-term response, but for many stress can be chronic in our modern society.

Actually, I was just reading an article the other day where all you need to do is look at pictures of sick people. Somewhere along the line in our evolution, seeing people who are sick puts our immune response on high alert.

Meditation is also thought to stimulate immune-system brain function regions, but it's not clear if this boost is just because it promotes a relaxed state of mind.

Having sex a couple times a week is ideal for immunity, with studies showing optimal IgA levels in the saliva.

http://www.onhealth.com/content/1/immune_system_boost

Pet owners often have lower blood pressure and triglyceride levels, which may translate to lower risks of heart disease.

Exercise, selective vitamins and foods are also well known to be a boost to the immune system.

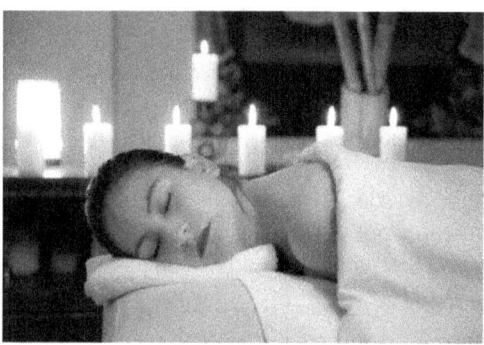

Stress, Anxiety, Depression and Panic Symptoms

Stressful situations are not necessarily the problem. Some people will thrive on a particular circumstance; others will tolerate it, while still others will struggle with it. Slamming on your breaks to avoid a collision is a stress response, should last moments, and should be easy to shake off, and everybody is built to tolerate these bursts of stress hormones.

However, stress means different things to different people. Stress was an evolutionary advantage in ancient times, with a gene that triggers the "fight" or "flight" syndrome, but for the most part, it's obsolete in today's modern society, unless you happen to be a mom who had an auto accident and is trying to get to her kids, and even then, these bursts of stress hormones serve their purpose, but we are just not built to handle extended periods of stress.

Stress is meant to be a short term response, but in modern society, people often experience periods of chronic stress, leading to a wide range of symptoms. Part of the problem is your body quickly breaks down proteins for the energy needed for fight or flight, so anyone who is chronically stressed needs to replenish these proteins frequently.

Chronic stress will inhibit the immune response, cardiovascular function, neuroendocrine function and central nervous system function, which can manifest itself in many ways for different people.

Medical studies have shown that the physical signs of stress contributes to overeating, belly fat, high blood pressure, headaches, migraines, stomachaches, diarrhea, constipation, insomnia, fatigue, irritability, restlessness, burnout, worry, tension, faintness, tingling, impatience, shaking, nail biting, fear, sweating, panic attacks, confusion, obsessive and intrusive thoughts, memory and concentration problems, anxious, anxiety, depression, strokes, heart disease, diabetes, colitis, asthma, rheumatism, skin allergies, sexual difficulties, hardening of the arteries, ulcers, breathing problems, kidney disorders, and weakening of the immune system, which can lead to a host of infections, chronic conditions and diseases.

Chronic stress is a serious condition and both directly and indirectly kills people. Stress is the polar opposite of relaxation, which is the state your body needs to rejuvenate and effectively fight disease. Stress suppresses many body functions that are not necessary for fight or flight, so things like the healing process just don't happen, with the exception of blood clotting for a wound.

Severe stress for any extended period of time can be physiologically and physiologically debilitating and can take a severe emotional toil with otherwise healthy individuals, so getting a handle on stress is the single best thing anyone can do for themselves, especially when fighting a disease.

Stress is the real underlying enemy for anyone who is coping with related symptoms, struggling with mental and physical health related conditions, allowing stress to affect everyday activities, trying to bounce-back from any disease and needs a well-functioning immune system, struggling with low energy, fatigue or burnout, or is just having difficulty maintaining their livelihood because of stress or related symptoms, or getting sick too frequently.

Fortunately, severe stress, often referred to as anxiety or depression, can be treatable with holistic approaches, nutrition, exercise, sleep, along with any combination of approaches covered in this book.

The great news is stress improvements can often be immediate, but will likely take some on-going effort to build up a strong tolerance and resilience, resulting in substantial improvements to overall health and wellbeing. It is all much easier and enjoyable than you might expect too, making stress manageable in a way that suites your lifestyle, instead of letting stress manage you, or even run you over.

Anything you can do to improve your overall health, and get a handle on stress, is also great for your immune system, making it harder to get sick, having more days where you feel on top of your game, and solving the underlying problem contributing to any challenge or condition you might be struggling with.

You found the right place for great answers to roll your own solution.

"When patience is needed, it's time to take action and throw yourself into your work or an enjoyable hobby, like reading a good book!" ~ Dan Harp

Overall Physical Stress, Anxiety and Panic Attack Relief

Perhaps the best way to think of stress, anxiety and panic attacks is "can you take a breath?", ok how about "can you take a deep breath?"

Because in the moment, that's really all you need to think about. Nothing else really matters and in the next moment, again all you need to concern yourself with is "can I take a breath?". Embrace this technique and make it your own. There is more information on breathing and pranayama under the toolbox section of this book.

Stretching is one of the best ways to relax quickly and feel at ease. Here's a good one that I picked up along the way that works really well. Find yourself a comfortable chair and follow along waiting 10 seconds between steps:

- Stretch your forehead
- Stretch your face
- Stretch your neck
- Stretch your upper body
- Stretch your arms
- Stretch your hands and fingers
- Stretch your back and abdomen

- Stretch your upper legs
- Stretch your lower legs
- Stretch your feet and toes
- Stretch your entire body

Now do the reverse at 5 seconds between steps:

- Stretch your feet and toes
- Stretch your lower legs
- Stretch your upper legs
- Stretch your back and abdomen
- Stretch your hands and fingers
- Stretch your arms
- Stretch your upper body
- Stretch your neck
- Stretch your face
- Stretch your forehead
- Stretch your entire body

My Doctors office has a poster in all the rooms. It says "if you could truly get the benefits of exercise in a pill, it would be the #1 selling supplements in the world".

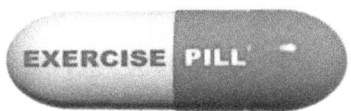

The Mayo Clinic recommends regular exercise for improved muscle strength, boost endurance, pump up the feel good endorphins in the brain, and improve mood, resulting in better metabolism, better night's sleep, better oxygen absorption, better nutrient absorption, more available energy and improved cardiovascular function.

Exercise is an excellent way to relieve stress and boost your immune system. When you get your heart pumping with aerobic exercise, your body releases serotonin and norepinephrine, which results in a feeling of euphoria and happiness, and helps to reduce pain.

A 20 minute workout is all it takes to reduce symptoms of stress, anxiety and depression, making you feel much calmer and happier.

There are many stretching exercises that you can do at your desk to reduce stress and boost energy.

Stress Exercises for Stress Relief
http://www.rd.com/health/wellness/stretching-exercises-for-stress-relief/

Stretching Exercises at Your Desk: 12 Simple Tips
http://www.webmd.com/fitness-exercise/stretching-exercises-at-your-desk-12-simple-tips

Desk Yoga: Stress-Relieving Back Stretches to do in Your Chair
http://life.gaiam.com/video/desk-yoga-stress-relieving-back-stretches-do-your-chair

Yoga incorporates breathing exercise, meditation, light exercise and energy flow that helps relieve stress. Greater practice brings greater resistance to stress. The "Wall Roll-Down", "Cat with a Twist:", and "Up the Wall", are very beneficial to reduce stress and maintain a good flow with your energy centers.

Sex can be an awesome stress reliever, which includes fun and effective techniques such as breathing, touching, social connection, rush of endorphins and beneficial chemical release with orgasm, all in one.

Overall Nutritional Stress Relief

Hunger and dehydration increase stress levels and elevated stress levels can lead to overeating for some people. Long term stress can cause continuous spikes in cortisol, insulin and ghrelin that increase appetite especially for fatty foods and sweet and salty comfort foods, which can increase the bodies overall stress levels.

Smaller portions of nutritional meals and fresh smoothies or healthy snacking will have immediate benefits making you resilient to stress.

The American Dietetic Association recommends a balanced diet including at least 5 servings of fruits and vegetables per day, which will help boost energy, combat diseases, improve mood and maintain a healthy metabolism for control weight.

A healthy balanced diet including lean meats, whole-grains, low-fat dairy products, and fresh fruits and vegetables, your body has the fuels that are needed to support healthy energy levels. You will also age better; fruits and vegetables are high in antioxidants that can help you protect your skin.

In particular, magnesium, antioxidants in berries and omega-3 fatty acids can prevent premature aging of skin cells and greatly help with stress.

Some of the best foods for reducing stress includes green leafy vegetables, asparagus, green tea, yogurt or other fermented foods, oatmeal, blueberries, pistachios, cashews, almonds, beef, turkey breast, wild salmon, tuna, dark chocolate, cottage cheese, seeds and fruits, especially oranges, pineapple, papaya, and cantaloupe for a quick boost of vitamin C.

An excellent superfood is beef bone broth soup loaded with collagen, which strengths your bones, cushions your joints, improves skin elasticity, improves adrenal function, improves hormonal balance, and reduces stress, also loaded with glycine which helps with liver detoxification and internally produced antioxidant availability, all very easy on the digestive system.

A healthy breakfast with complex carbohydrates helps the body sustain energy throughout the day, so don't skip the most important meal of the day, Carbohydrates release serotonin, a feel-good neurotransmitter in the brain that will help you feel more calm and collective as you start your day.

Eat a healthy snack between meals to refuel and ensure that blood sugar levels don't drop. This includes protein to boost energy and healthy fat to help maintain it over time. Balancing proteins and healthy fat for meals will increase the burn for high energy and help with weight loss.

Avocados provide about 20 essential health-boosting nutrients. Those who eat a half of an avocado for lunch report being hunger free for hours, while maintaining healthy blood sugar levels, and a steady mood even at time of stress, all without snacking.

Drink plenty of water to help burn calories and fat for energy and stave fatigue.

Processed foods have a long list of mood-busting ingredients including trans fats, monosodium glutamate (MSG), artificial sweeteners, sugar, gluten and much more.

Gluten found in wheat inhibits the production of serotonin, resulting in depression, because of WGA - Wheat Germ Agglutinin results in neurotoxic activity.

Stress consumes resources at a much quicker rate than normal, so proper nutrition is very important at times of stress. The better choice is proteins and healthy fats, or some of the above superfoods for stress relief.

Vitamin, Mineral and Amino Acid Stress and Depression Relief

Some foods will help moderate the body's levels of cortisol, the stress hormone. Foods packed with magnesium, omega 3-fatty acids, and vitamin C will reduce cortisol levels.

Ancient Minerals – Magnesium Benefits
http://www.ancient-minerals.com/magnesium-benefits/

Folic Acid will help as a natural anti-depressant and prevents depression. It is also known to help prevent heart disease, type-2 diabetes, Alzheimer's and some forms of cancer. It helps the body breakdown, create and use new proteins. It is synergetic with Vitamin B-12 as a coenzyme to help metabolism.

Supplement up to 450 mcl daily or simply eat plenty of dark green vegetables instead. Excessive supplementation of folic acid can interact with rubbing alcohol and bronchitis/smoking and result in eczema and COPD. I can only guess what kind of interactions might occur with drinking alcohol. In any case, discontinuing the folic acid along with what it is interacting with, should reverse the condition in as little as a few weeks.

Shots of vitamin B-12 are the most efficient way to absorb this essential nutrient. B-12 deficiency is more common than doctors admit. Resolving this deficiency will help improve energy levels, increase metabolic rate of proteins and fats, improve mood, regulate sleep, and improve appetite. Al fat soluble toxic chemicals require B-12 to be cleansed by your liver, so this vitamin is essential for toxic overload.

Vitamin B Complex will help fight fatigue and also speeds up your metabolism. These vitamins help keep your body running like a well-oiled machine by converting food in to fuel, allowing us to be energized throughout the day. Most people's healthy diets already have enough of these vitamins, but B-12 in particular can be depleted especially with vegans and the elderly. It is possible to take too much B-3 and B-6 vitamins, so be careful of complex dosages.

Vitamin C helps protect the immune system and helps reduce cortisol levels. It is essential for improved cardiac health, protecting against cancer, speeds the clearance of stomach disease-causing bacterium, shortens the duration of common colds, reduces the risk of serious repertory conditions, helps avoid degenerative diseases, supports healthy blood sugar levels in diabetes, dramatically reduces oxidative damage in the body and enhances the health-promoting effects of exercise.

With Vitamin D, a simple blood test at your doctors will tell you everything you need to know. Low levels of this important nutrient can result in many symptoms, lead to many diseases, and can be an indication of poor health is in the works.

The parathyroid gland which regulates vitamin D is not particularly smart. It draws both vitamin D and calcium at the same time, so if vitamin D is deficient, it will keep trying, so excessive calcium is continuously drawn from the bones, which acts as a reservoir for calcium.

This excessive calcium needs to be excreted or reabsorbed, but most people's intake of calcium is often too high to begin with, so calcium starts building up in soft tissue resulting in hardening and calcification.

Vitamin D is also considered protective against many diseases such as osteoporosis, osteopenia, osteoarthritis, heart disease, schizophrenia, erectile dysfunction, infertility, obesity, 17 forms of cancer including aggressive prostate cancer, fibromyalgia, Alzheimer disease, dementia, to name a few, which could ultimately lead to death.

Vitamin D is a common deficiency and can result in bone, joint, muscle and chronic pain, which are some of the many symptoms, along with weak bones and teeth, hypertension, tiredness, psoriasis, and chronic infections.

This important nutrient is often obtained from the sun, but is found in egg yolk, salmon, shrimp and sardines and is fortified in foods such as milk, cereal, yogurt, and orange juice, but when that's not enough, or glandular problems exist, supplementation is necessary.

This vitamin is important for the regulation of calcium and phosphorus absorption, needed for healthy bones and teeth, helps support the immune system, brain and nervous function, helps support lung function and cardiovascular function and even reduces the chance of getting the flu.

Studies have shown that people with low levels of vitamin D were many times more prone to depression than those who received healthy doses.

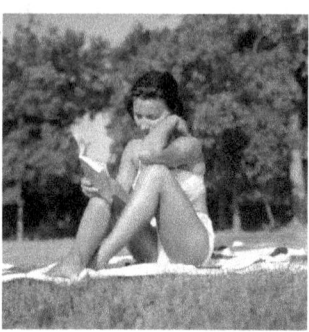

Sunshine will also stabilize your mood by raising serotonin levels in the brain, in addition to increased Vitamin D levels.

Take between 500 to 1,000 mg of L-Tyrosine to increase the production of dopamine and norepinephrine, making you more alert.

If you are stressed for any length of time, visit your primary care physician and have them check for any vitamin deficiencies that might be contributing to your stress. This is usually covered by insurance.

If you are fighting a disease, do some homework on what vitamins, minerals, amino acids and herbs can help as part of your tool belt. Don't rely on a single multivitamin. Get what you want in individual containers, so you can try them separately and have more control over the dosage.

In time, this will allow you to assess what you need each morning depending on how well you have been eating, how active you have been, how well you are feeling and of course what you are craving.

Benefits of Minerals 101

http://www.fitnesshealth101.com/fitness/nutrition/vitamins-minerals/mineral-benefits

Vitamin Glossary 101
http://www.fitnesshealth101.com/nutritional-glossary/vitamin

Amino Acid Glossary 101
http://www.fitnesshealth101.com/nutritional-glossary/amino-acid

Herb Glossary 101
http://www.fitnesshealth101.com/nutritional-glossary/herb

The Ultimate Guide to Vitamins and Minerals
http://greatist.com/health/ultimate-guide-vitamins-and-minerals

Consult your local health store. They are usually very friendly and knowledgeable. While you are there, ask them what they think about stress formulas such as Nerve Tonic and Sedalia. I can already tell you that Noni Juice is really good for stress and liver function, but haven't tried the other two.

Top Stress Busting and Depression Superfoods

Smoothie preparations often include ingredients that are healthy and delicious that can be effective for stress relief, but here is a list of superfood smoothie ingredients that you can't go wrong with against stress, for your healthy recipes and delicious smoothies. You can find a free coupon at the back of this book for a free eBook on delicious smoothie recipes.

Stressful situations are often unavoidable, but something as simple as an occasional smoothie can make all the difference in the world to how well you hold up to stressful situations, and how well you rebound from stress, so your immune system doesn't become impaired by stress, and you don't find yourself sick as a result of being over stressed.

Treat yourself to these nutritious creamy rich delicious easy "stress busting" smoothie ingredients, for a breakfast smoothie, or in any healthy recipe, and fill your body with loads of nutrients, including protein, vitamins, minerals, amino acids and enzymes for stress relief, to build your resilience to stress, and to calm your frazzled nerves.

Stress is the polar opposite of the deep relaxing, delta wave rest state needed for rejuvenation and a well-functioning immune system. A healthy and delicious smoothie will hit the spot and could easily complement anything else you might be doing, including coping with challenges and conditions like stress, anxiety and depression.

Bananas have potassium, which helps regulate blood pressure at times of stress, along with manganese and Vitamin B6, which helps produce serotonin, the happiness and feel good hormone.

Flaxseed is a powerhouse of nutrition, with Omega-3 essential oils which reduce stress, along with protein which helps to replenish depleted resources from stress. It offers so many benefits against cancer, diabetes, cholesterol, blood pressure, digestion, asthma, arthritis, and inflammation.

Mangos are known as the "King of Fruit", contains the linalool compound which has antidepressant and anti-anxiety effects, protects against cancer, diabetes and strokes, prevents early ageing and degenerative disease, improves eye health, lowers cholesterol and triglycerides, improves immunity, improves skin health, and improves digestion.

Blueberries have anthocyanins that increase production of dopamine in the brain, a chemical critical to coordination, memory function, and your mood.

Fruits high in antioxidants and Vitamin CA and are recognized as stress reducing by lowering cortisol levels. Studies have shown that fruits and vegetables of any kind help calm the nerves, feeling calmer, happier and more energetic.

Yogurt eases stress, anxiety and depression, by blocking emotion and pain and help keep a "feel good" state of mind. Probiotics can change the makeup of your gut flora making you more stress resilient.

Coconut Oil is often considered more effective than drugs at combating stress and depression. **Coconut water** contains minerals that help to rebalance electrolyte levels to help keep you calm.

Dark Chocolate provides a mood burst, increasing anandamide, a brain neurotransmitter that blocks pain, anxiety and depression, along with other chemicals that prolong the "feel-good" aspects of anandamide. It is very nutritious, loaded with antioxidants, helps lower blood pressure, raises HDL, protects LDL from oxidation, and may lower the risk of cardiovascular disease.

Peanut Butter makes you less likely to develop heart related issues or type-2 diabetes, despite the sugar and fat content, and it's a great source of protein which is necessary to replenish at times of stress.

Spinach is loaded with magnesium, which helps with general fatigue, along with folate, which helps your body produce mood-regulating neurotransmitters.

Kale is very high in vitamins, minerals and antioxidants that are effective for stress, liver function, prevention of cancer and Alzheimer's, is an effective anti-inflammatory, supports the cardivascular system, vision, skin, immune system, and metabolism, and is a great detox food because of the high sulfur and fiber content.

Seeds, nuts, green leafy vegetables like spinach, seaweed, avocados and Swiss chad are all excellent sources of magnesium, which is well known for numerous benefits, including reduced anxiety, panic attacks, depression, fatigue, and headaches, improves sleep and helps regulate serotonin, energy, emotions, and wellbeing.

Vegetables that are particularly good for stress relief includes kale, spinach, seaweed, broccoli, beet, asparagus, cabbage, and cilantro.

Pomegranate lowers the stress hormone cortisone, improves memory, has impressive anti-inflammatory effects, helps lower blood pressure, helps fight cancer, arthritis and joint pain, bacterial infections and fungal infections, and lowers your risk of heart disease.

Avocados have about 20 essential health-boosting nutrients, helps curb appetite, helps regulate blood sugar levels, is a good source of magnesium, and helps to keep your mood steady, even at times of stress.

Ginger helps to boost your mood and clear out chemicals secreted by the body that leads to stress from being worried.

Vanilla bean helps calm, soothe, and relax the body and its smell activates the feel-good sensations in the brain.

Cinnamon improves mood, alertness, memory, brain function and depression, helps control blood sugar levels, digestion, IBS – Irritable Bowel Syndrome, weight loss, cholesterol, triglycerides, and is an antioxidant, antibacterial, antimicrobial, and even helps fight stomach bugs, flu, cold, E-coli, sore throat, cough, salmonella, and candida yeast infections. It also helps prevent cancer, arthritis, osteoporosis, Alzheimer's disease, Parkinson's disease, and gum disease.

A special mention to **milk chocolate**; recent studies show it to be good for the heart, reducing both heart disease and strokes. It is rich in antioxidants and magnesium, but is high in calories. Even so, two bars a day may be at least as good for you as dark chocolate, as a boost to your brain, libido and even your figure, along with improved memory, hydrating your skin and even boosting your immune system.

Not such a guilty pleasure after all, right!

Holistic Approach to Severe Stress, Anxiety and Depression Relief

Many of us simply don't like doctors, usually from experience, often because of concern that they are useless at coming up with a treatment for you, concern about what they might find, concern about having a diagnosed physiological disorder, concern about pharmaceuticals and their side effects, or all of the above.

Even so, if your symptoms get out of control, any decent doctor should be able to prescribe something that can help for stress, anxiety and depression, even if you prefer to consider it temporary to hold you over.

Fortunately, severe stress often referred to as anxiety or depression, can be treatable with a holistic approach using natural herbs, amongst the many tips and techniques you will find throughout. Herbal treatments have been around for centuries and are widely used across the world even today.

Chamomile is often used in tea or infusion, but is available in a liquid extract, as a capsule, or even as a mouthwash. It is often used as a relaxing beverage before bedtime, and serves as a sleeping aid. Medical studies have shown it to substantially reduce systems of stress and anxiety over time.

Green Tea (L-theanine) amino acid allows Buddhist monks to meditate for hours while being both alert and relaxed. This amino acid lowers blood pressure, regulates heart rate, and reduces stress and anxiety. This is one you can take without making you drowsy. This amino acid is available in supplement form, allowing you to get the equivalent of several cups of tea.

Lemon Balm has been used since the middle ages for stress and anxiety relief and acts as a sleeping aid. Medical studies have shown healthy individuals taking it were more calm and alert. It is often taken as a tea or in capsule form, but follow directions, excessive doses can heighten anxiety.

St. John's Wort has been medically proven for stress relief and mild depression, and is at least effective against some stress related symptoms, taken in extract and capsule forms, but the holistic community recommends it for a number of remedies.

Kava Kava is also a sleeping aid that helps with restlessness. It is often used as a tea or infusion and is also available in capsule form. In Hawaii, it has traditionally been used as a treatment for Asthma.

Passionflower is cure for stress and restlessness, actually a remedy for many conditions, often regarded as one of those miracle cures. It is most often consumed in tea and as dry leaves or orally. Side effects can occur when taken with other drugs, so do some research or consult your doctor.

Lavender is often used for aromatherapy for anxiety and restfulness, and is generally not taken orally. There are a few potential side effects that can be avoided if you have your doctor check you out first.

Hops, in extract form, not in your beer, are an effective sedative to help with stress and for a restful night's sleep. This herb shouldn't be taken with prescriptions that act as sedatives or tranquilizers, so do some research or consult your doctor for drug interactions.

Valerian is a sleeping aid for insomnia that acts as a sedative. Because of the odor, most people take it in capsule form. It is often combined with other sedative herbs like hops, chamomile, and lemon balm.

Probiotics Stress Relief

Probiotics support the trillions of "good" bacteria that live on the inner walls of your large intestines, which fight harmful bacteria, help with your mood and emotional response to stress, reduces anxiety, depression and memory loss and helps with the digestion of fiber making vitamins B and K.

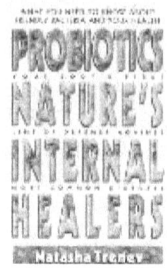

Probiotics: Nature's Internal Healers by Natasha Trenev includes an A-Z list of illnesses and disorders that can be prevented or corrected with proper probiotic supplementation. Probiotics – the friendly bacteria that reside in you gastrointestinal tract are your body's first line of defense against the potentially harmful microorganisms you inhale or ingest. Natasha Trenev explains the importance of these bacteria in achieving and maintaining good health.

Possibly the two most beneficial bacteria to have are Lactobacillus and Bifidobacterium. These can increase tryptophan in the blood, which is a precursor to the feel good neurotransmitters serotonin and dopamine. The stress hormone norepinephrine promotes well known pathogens like Escherichia Coli, causing diarrhea, so "good" bacteria can prevent that.

Alkaline Balance Stress Relief

Alkaline foods can help with detoxification, reduces stress and improves your overall energy. Acidic foods draw alkaline nutrients and minerals from the body to neutralize the effect, which can lead to a buildup of acids in the cells and further calcification. Diseases favor an acidic state, so with the onslaught of acidity from stress and diet, balance is needed to maintain health and more focus on your alkaline intake is needed to fight disease.

Human blood pH should be somewhat alkaline between 7.35 and 7.45. Anything below or above this range suggests symptoms of disease. A pH balance of 7.00 is neutral, below that is acidic and above that is alkaline. Common causes of acidity include toxic overload, stress, and immune reactions that deprive the cells of oxygen and ability to absorb nutrients and minerals.

Diets consisting of 50% alkaline forming foods are recommended to maintain health. To restore health and promote decalcification of the pineal gland, diets of at least 75% alkaline are suggested.

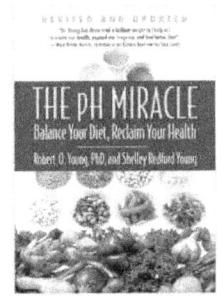

Dr. Robert Young book: The pH Miracle: Balance Your Diet, Reclaim Your Health, explains why you should never count calories, fat grams, or portion sizes ever again. The body's pH balance is the key to optimal weight, mental clarity, and overall vigor. Say good-by to low energy, poor digestion, extra-pounds, aches and pains, and disease.

Complete coverage of core nutrients, cleansing, exercising right, and alkaline foods.

Although many fruits are acidic, most are actually alkaline-forming in the body.

Amongst the best alkaline forming foods to eat are fresh fruits, green vegetables, nuts and seeds.

Highly alkaline forming foods include baking soda, lime, lemons, lentils, lotus root, mineral water, nectarine, onion, persimmon, pineapple, pumpkin seed, raspberry, sea salt, sea vegetables, seaweed, sweet potato, tangerine and watermelon. Fresh lemonade and watermelon are particularly effective for detoxification of the pineal gland.

Alkaline based homemade smoothies and juices are highly effective.

Raw Apple Cider Vinegar is rich is malic acid and helps alkalize the body, it's a great way to detoxify and decalcify the body. You can have it straight up or with a glass of water, lemon juice, honey, tea or as a salad dressing. For best results, take before meals, anywhere from 1 to 3 teaspoons, 1 to 2 times daily, when choosing a brand, make sure it is in a bottle rather than plastic, raw, organic and has "The Mother" in it.

Extremely acidic foods include alcohol, artificial sweeteners, beef, beer, breads, brown sugar, carbonated soft drinks, cereals , chicken, chocolate, cigarettes, coffee, custard, deer, eggs, fish, flour, fruit juices with sugar, grains, jams, jellies, lamb, maple syrup (processed), meats, pasta (white), white flour, pickles (commercial), pork, seafood, sugar (white), table salt (refined and iodized), tea (black), turkey, white bread, white vinegar (processed), whole wheat foods, wine, and yogurt (sweetened).

Acidic fruits are blueberries, canned fruits, glazed fruits, cranberries, currants, plums, and prunes.

Acidic vegetables are corn, lentils, olives and winter squash.

Acidic nuts include cashews, legumes, peanut butter, peanuts, pecans, tahini, and walnuts.

There are a wide range of resources on the internet to review alkaline foods and recipes.

Alkaline Food Lists
https://www.google.com/search?q=alkaline+foods+list

Alkaline Food Recipes
https://www.google.com/search?q=Alkaline+Food+Recipes

You can also do wonders for your wellbeing with homemade juices and smoothies, which is covered throughout.

Vices in Moderation

Americans get the most antioxidants in their diet from coffee. I personally love my java, but thought this radio fact was funny, mostly because I've been guilty and because I know there are so many other great sources of antioxidants.

Caffeine helps to amplify stress throughout the day, both in terms of stress hormone levels and blood pressure elevations, according to the National Instates of Health.

Many doctors and commercials these days blame smoking for all of the world's problems. Actually, smoking has benefits of reducing stress and tension while boosting mood and creativity, especially if you drink caffeinated coffee, which is like balancing your "Chi", which loosely translates to "Energy" on the physical plane. Neither is particularly good for you in the long term, but together it works, like "Yin" and "Yang", if you believe two wrongs can make a right.

Make no mistake that stress is the root cause of more health related problems than smoking, caffeine and all other factors combined, except for maybe Vitamin D deficiency, although there are those that would argue anything that can contribute to stress is the root cause of stress, but that argument is like saying life is the root cause of stress.

Having said that, everyone has different tolerance levels... I can personally drink many triple-shot coffees and eat chocolate covered coffee beans at levels that have given the java jitters to others who have tried to keep up. If you feel caffeine is contributing to your stress, or coffee is making you feel dehydrated, which also contributes to stress, you can always cut down on coffee, drink more water during the day, switch to decaffeinated coffee, or try a half caffeinated and half decaffeinated blend.

Coffee also has a wide range of studied benefits:

- Increases your fiber intake
- Protects against cirrhosis of the liver
- Lowers risk of type 2 diabetes
- Lowers risk of Alzheimer disease
- Helps prevent heart disease
- Reduces risk of suicide with depression
- Protects against Parkinson's
- Reduces muscle pain from workouts
- Stronger DNA integrity
- Reduces liver cancer risk
- Less risk of Gout
- Longevity
- Minerals (including calcium and magnesium)
- Vitamins (including vitamin B2 and B5)

Honey is one of the oldest sweeteners on earth and has many studied benefits, including:

- Helps regulate blood sugar
- Reduces cough and throat irritation
- Improves athletic performance
- Is both anti-bacterial and anti-fungal
- Is a probiotic
- Helps with ulcers and gastrointestinal trouble
- Helps prevent cancer
- Helps prevent heart disease
- Helps improve the skin
- Antioxidants
- Minerals (including calcium, iron, magnesium, phosphate, potassium, sodium chlorine and sulphur)
- Vitamins (including vitamin B1, B2, B3, B5, B6 and C)

The sugars in honey are sweeter, so you don't need as much, and they burn faster, so they are less likely to be converted to fat, and will have less of an effect on blood-glucose levels.

For some people, honey has a stronger flavor that doesn't always go well with coffee, but the idea it to use less, so it might be worth a try.

If doctors were paid based on how well they performed, or how well their service actually helped you, they wouldn't be coming up with excuses, like asking if you smoke or drink caffeine, they would be asking you if you felt stressed instead, and how often are you stressed?

Smoking does however have its problems too, similar to not eating right, or not getting enough exercise, or not getting enough sleep, or abusing certain substances. Stress can lead to elevated smoking that can in turn contribute to making you more nervous and stressed. The real problem though is people who smoke, and those who are coping with conditions and diseases, often don't get enough exercise, along with all of the benefits of higher levels of activity can bring.

Smoking can also deplete Vitamin C levels, which can reduce your tolerance to stress, and make you more susceptible to colds, but supplementation of Vitamin C will help with that.

Everybody has different tolerances and there are definitely people who shouldn't smoke. For people trying to rebound from a disease, don't be too hard on yourself if you can't or don't want to quit smoking, but consider a balanced approach, maybe a more nutritious diet, detoxing, cleansing, smoothies or juicing, and understand that stress is the real enemy, not smoking.

The VaporFi Vice is a great substation for smoking or at least helps at times when you can't smoke. The Trixler (Raspberry and Passion Fruit) flavor is really good too.

Look at it this way, in a few hundred years it won't matter much anyway. People at that time will probably be sitting back enjoying an occasional smoke or joint, talking about the 21st century as if it were still part of the "Dark Ages of Medicine", while drinking down their caffeinated coffee.

Some say "Feed a Cold and Starve a Fever" while others say 'Feed a Fever and Starve a Cold'. What's easier to remember is "Drown a Cold and Drown a Fever"… An occasional night out with good friends and your favorite cocktails or IPA bears can work wonders for making you relaxed and stress free. The problem with going overboard is heavy alcohol use acts as a depressant by slowing down the neurotransmitters in the brain that are needed for good mental health, which in turn will increase stress.

Stress Management Tips and Techniques

Physical activity, a healthy diet, and a good night's rest are all helpful at reducing stress. Try getting as much as 8-9 hours of uninterrupted sleep at night. If insomnia is part of the problem, you can try some natural remedies that include Melatonin or herbs that act as sedatives.

Although laughter may not be the easiest thing to do when you are stressed, it is one of the best medicines for stress symptoms. It reduces stress hormone levels, releases tension and brings positive physiological changes, so hit a comic club, watch your favorite sitcom, do a prank, or do whatever gets a laugh out of you.

Breathing exercises are immediately beneficial. Simply take a deep breath from your diaphragm, slowly through your noise, while your belly expands, exhale slowly and repeat a few times. Slow deep breathing with long deep breathes serves to relax the nervous system.

Heating up the body with a warm bath, sun bathing, warm fire, sauna, steam room, or even a hot cup of tea, will reduce muscle tension and anxiety and makes you more relaxed and improves mood, including serotonin release.

Listening to music can be a great way to relax and help with stress, has a calming effect while facing the day's stressors, but choose music that already resonates with you, that you already know will lift your spirits and help you get back into the groove.

Take a forest bath, known as Skinrin-yoku by the Japanese, which more accurately translates to a short walk in the woods with all the outdoor odors and background sounds of streams, proven to reduce stress hormone levels and make you more relaxed in no time.

Relieve tension and stress by applying pressure to your pressure points. Simply breathe deeply and apply steady pressure for a few minutes. Common pressure points to do include the temples, the point between both eyebrows, the back of the neck slightly below the scull, about an inch down from your shoulders, towards the back of your neck, or anywhere you feel aching when you apply pressure.

Mantras are an excellent way to silence the self-critical voice that can result with stress. Try coming up with a manta of the day, or just as needed, as part of your routine mental exercise. Simple mantras might go something like "I'm Ready for This" or "Bring it". Repeat your manta of the day at least several times, with several successions. The Ahh meditation technique or even staring at a burning candle serves to relax the mind, allow focus, and reduce stress symptoms.

Enjoy aromatherapy for stress relief, to become more energized, relaxed and present. Lavender is associated with feelings of contentment, cognitive performance, and mood. Peppermint is particularly good for stress, memory and alertness and is a great pick-me-up. Vanilla Extract is often readily available and is very uplifting for your mood. Basil, hay, eucalyptus, rose, and thyme oils are also very soothing.

You can do acupuncture too, it has been proven to reduce stress hormone levels. I've never tried it personally, but my sister swears by it and some insurance companies will pay for it.

Massage therapy feels great and is a very popular way to relax and relieve stress, preferably a full body massage.

Get yourself a great life coach who is really in the now like Kidest OM. If anyone can get you out of a funk, she can, and then some; she is very inspirational.

Kidest OM on YouTube
https://www.youtube.com/results?search_query=Kidest+OM

EMT – Emotional Freedom Technique is a form of physical acupressure that is based on the energy meridians used in acupuncture to treat physical and emotional ailments for over five thousand years.

It can help your body eliminate emotional "scarring" and the way you respond to emotional stressors. It helps reduce negative emotions, reduce food cravings, reduce or eliminate pain and helps you implement positive goals.

EMT – Emotional Freedom Technique
http://eft.mercola.com/

PMR – Progressive Muscle Relaxation is a technique that lets you relax all the muscles in your body in groups. It only takes several minutes and lets you feel physically and emotionally relaxed. With practice, it can be done in seconds.

PMR – Progressive Muscle Relaxation
http://stress.about.com/od/stressmanagementglossary/g/pmr.htm

Do something you enjoy, like a hobby, crafts, art, dancing, volunteer work, etc. Enjoy a good game with friends or play something relaxing to take your mind off of stressors.

Gardening can be a great stress reliever. It combines satisfaction for your creation with exercise and getting outside in the sun and enjoying the scenery.

Do something active like a sport, including racket ball, swimming, basketball, volleyball, skiing, or just take a long walk, etc. These can all be fantastic stress relievers that get you in a different frame of mind and work in minutes.

Playing with and caring for pets are a great way to help you focus on the moment.

Roll with the punches and when you get the opportunity to be proactive, take it. Don't let yourself become a victim or feel helpless, that's the true path to the dark side, stress.

Did you know that loneliness and social isolation are twice as dangerous as obesity for mortality? Make a point to get together with family and friends. A lifestyle that allows you to feel safe, secure, empowered or important makes you more resilient to stress.

Accept that there are circumstances beyond your control, so there is no point aimlessly dwelling on them.

Maintain a positive attitude and outlook, don't let yourself be pessimistic.

Takes 15 minute breaks when you feel overwhelmed, to relax and reflect. Learn relaxation techniques like meditation, yoga and breathing.

There are psychologists who specialize in stress management. In many cases, some forms of antidepressants can help manage the symptoms, but you may need to work on what is causing you to be overwhelmed with your current situation, along with addressing any underlying emotional, behavioral or lifestyle causes, to fully get back to normal function.

Mindfulness Meditation Stress Relief

Mindfulness meditation was originally a Buddhist practice that is very effective in stress and anxiety relief. All you do is practice paying attention to the present moment, with curiosity and nonjudgmental observation.

Practicing mindful awareness allows you to focus on each moment as it occurs, which is not necessarily how you would perceive it otherwise, if it catches your attention at all.

The act of focusing on something other than your worries alone will take you out of the "stress" zone, and help put you in the "now" zone.

Try to focus on how your breath feels coming in and out of your body. Try some breathing exercises too and take notice of the change. Ask yourself simple questions about what you are experiencing in the moment, like: Does your breath feel different as it enters or exits your body? How does a deeper breath feel differently?

Mindfulness technique is all about consciously being aware of your focus while living the moment, rather than letting your mind wonder aimlessly at times of stress and anxiety.

Another good use of your focus is to smile. This comes natural when you are relaxed and happy, but doing it when you're not will cause your facial muscles to stimulate a sense of calmness.

Another good use of your focus is stop slumping, a common symptom of stress, which restricts your breathing and reduces blood and oxygen flow to your brain, contributes to muscle tension and a sense of panic, so straitening your back and maintaining a good posture has the opposite effect, reducing your stress levels.

Even becoming aware of your emotional state or physiological responses to stress is a great use of your focus, and a great first step in reducing your stress and anxiety levels. This book provides many tools for your tool belt, so the next step is to pull out the tool(s) of choice and observe, in the moment, the level of improvement, until eventually, you have it all on autopilot.

Relaxation and Visualization Meditation Stress Relief

Meditation has been practiced in the East for centuries and is becoming more popular in the western cultures. It causes relaxation that lowers the heart rate, blood pressure, breathing, stress hormone levels, and relieves anxiety.

As Hugh Jackson put it, "Meditation is all about the pursuit of nothingness. It's like the ultimate rest. It's better than the best sleep you've ever had. It's a quieting of the mind. It sharpens everything, especially your appreciation of your surroundings. It keeps life fresh"

Meditation for 30 minutes a day has been shown to reduce stress hormones by as much as 25%. People who practiced Buddhist meditations "Om" daily for 6 weeks significantly reduced both cortisol hormone levels and blood pressure.

The primary benefits of meditation include reduced stress, inflammation, lower blood pressure, reduced anxiety, headaches, insomnia, and tension, lower risk of ulcers, improved mood, emotional strength, expands intuition, focus, calmness, concentration, and boosts immune system and energy levels.

Relaxation meditation is the simplest form of meditation. It's probably best to start out with guided meditations and move on to background music with your own mantras. It's a skill you will get better at with practice, allowing you to recognize your true nature and being that already exists in you, a higher state of thoughtless awareness, ultimately allowing you to take greater control.

Try some Guided Meditations for Stress too
https://www.youtube.com/results?search_query=Guided+Meditation+Stress

YouTube is an Excellent Source for Relaxation Meditation
https://www.youtube.com/results?search_query=Reaxation+Meditation

Visualization mediation is the next most difficult form of meditation, which allows you to utilize visualization and mental imagery to promote relaxation of mind and body.

As David Lynch put it "Meditation is to dive all the way within, beyond thought, to the source of thought and pure consciousness. It enlarges the container, every time you transcend. When you come out, you come out refreshed, filled with energy and enthusiasm for life".

Step up to some Visualization Meditations
https://www.youtube.com/results?search_query=Visualization+Meditations

Self-hypnosis Stress Relief Techniques

You can find seminars to manage the stress in your life. One helpful self-hypnosis technique that I picked up many years ago at a stress seminar goes something like this...

Feel free to adopt it and make it your own. Just find yourself a comfortable place, follow along with a similar dialog while visualizing that you are actually there in the moment.

Other forms of meditation are covered at the end of this book, under the section called "Power Tools for your Tool Belt".

- You find yourself on the roof top of a ten story building
- You walk towards an elevator door as it opens for you
- You enter and push the button for the first floor; your eyelids get heavier and heavier
- As you approach the ninth floor, you take a deep breath and release it slowly
- As you reach the eighth floor, you find yourself getting very relaxed
- As you reach the seventh floor, you are getting even more relaxed
- As you reach the sixth floor, you are feeling very comfortable and relaxed
- As you reach the firth floor, the door opens and all your concerns, worries and tensions float away through the halls of the fifth floor.
- As the door closes, you know you are leaving everything behind you
- You approach the fourth floor, feeling better than ever
- You approach the third four with a very deep relaxation
- You approach the second floor in a deeper state of relaxation
- You approach the first floor, completely relaxe
- On the first floor, the doors open to a sandy beach.
- You step out and feel the warm sand though your toes
- You feel the sun shining on you, making you warm and comfortable.
- You hear the roar of the ocean with the waves crashing on the beach

- You smell the salt air and feel cool breeze
- As you look around, you see something close to the beach on the horizon
- As you get closer, it looks like a pyramid
- You walk closer and closer until you see an open door
- As you reach the door, you see a long hallway with a blue light at the end
- You enter the pyramid; go down the hallway, to a large open chamber
- As you enter the chamber, you can feel the residency vibrations of the earth being amplified throughout the room
- This frequency and vibration runs through you and around you, embracing you until your entire body resonates with the earth.
- You feel your body rejuvenating and healing itself
- You feel your body cleansing itself
- You feel your body renewing itself
- You realize this is your beach and your pyramid and your chamber and your earth and you can go anywhere anytime.
- The earth continues to vibrate through you and around you
- You feel it more and more as your body becomes completely rejuvenated and revitalized
- You walk back to the beach, towards the building you came from
- You see a blanket on the beach and decide to laydown
- You feel the warmth of the sun as your body tans to its touch
- You feel the suns energy flowing through you and around you
- You are in perfect harmony with the earth and the sun
- You go into the ocean to cool off.
- The salt water is so refreshing and rejuvenating
- You let the sun dry you as you head back to the building you came in on
- As you approach the building, the elevator doors open
- You enter the elevator and push the button for the tenth floor
- As you approach the second floor, you feel very refresh
- As you approach the third floor, you feel even more refreshed
- As you approach the fourth floor, you feel completely rejuvenated
- As you approach the fifth floor, you feel complete rejuvenated
- As you approach the sixth floor, you start feeling awake and alert
- As you approach the seventh you feel more awake and alert
- As you approach the eight you feel wide awake and alert
- As you approach the ninth you feel all around great
- As you reach the tenth floor, the door and eyes opens as you step out on the roof top

Stress is an Energy Vampire

Vibrational Energy Influences

Several years ago I was working for an Aerospace & Defense company in the former "Plastics Capital of the World". I was on a six month project in El Segundo, California. The change of scenery, sunshine, great food, great sites, working hard and playing harder seemed to really be agreeing with me.

Once I got back to my normal routine, I was noticing something strange. The week started out feeling great, with a steady decline during the week and by the weekend I had to mostly crash just to rebound.

I was noticing my desk had a vibration to it, presumably from the air compressors on the roof, but my audio and video equipment wasn't sensitive enough to record it. I asked around and found out a couple of my co-workers were experiencing the same kind of thing, but they were somewhat scarred to report it.

I already had a couple of outstanding claims for being exposed to hazardous chemicals in incidents that the company was try to cover up, do I had nothing to lose in complaining about this.

I didn't stop there. My thought was to fight fire with fire. If low frequency sound could make you feel lousy and run-down, the right kind of sound could be uplifting and make you feel great, alert, calm and collective.

So after some quick research, I came across what I was looking for on YouTube, quickly realized it worked, and shared some of it with my co-workers...

You will need a headset for some of these...

Magic Healing Music – With Frequencies of Rejuvenation
https://www.youtube.com/results?search_query=Magic+Healing+Music

10 Minute Rejuvenation with Alpha Brainwave Rejuvenation
https://www.youtube.com/results?search_query=10+Minute+Rejuvenation

Inner Bliss and Harmony – Isochoric Beats
https://www.youtube.com/results?search_query=Inner+Bliss+and+Harmony

Twilight Relaxation Binaural Beats
https://www.youtube.com/results?search_query=+Twilight+Relaxation+Binaural+Beats

After years of studying technologies to listen to brainwave frequencies, their benefits and application, I was convinced that these technologies could be put to use in a way that would have huge market potential for advanced learning, relaxation, rejuvenation, accelerated healing, awakening of the mind, self-reprograming of the mind, virtual prescriptions for diseases, entertainment value, and even as harmless recreational drugs.

The best part about this field of study is that none of it is regulated. Combined with other techniques and technologies, such as software that lets you do your own subliminal programing, the possibilities are limitless.

I experimented with creating my own works, but mostly just enjoyed the works of others and put them to good use. The bottom line is it would be very difficult to get the funding for projects and research to do this kind of work without the proper credentials.

The brain produces different brainwaves based on mood and stimuli which can be measured on an EEG machine, in the form of Hertz (cycles per second).

There is always a predominate brainwave that determines the homonym brain state.

In time these technologies will advance to the point where a single video curriculum will achieve the results you are looking for. In the meantime, you pretty much need to create an IPod mix of many works and listen to them frequently, or even take a shock-and-awe approach to awaken your mind.

Music and sound can be a very powerful transitional tool for your body and mind, but popular modern day music is not usually done at the scale that our ancestors used for healing, activating their minds, and transformation of the mind body. Modern day music is slightly out of scale, using a 440 Hz, which was changed from 417 Hz in 1914. The vocal scale was changed to "DO, RE, MI, FA, SO, LA, TI" from the original scale of "UT, RE, MI, FA, SO, LA".

The principle here is like striking a tuning fork or musical triangle and holding it next to another, just to observe it resonate too. This is similar to what happens when you listen to frequencies and brainwave entrainment, which coaxes the brain to synchronize.

Today's scientists are now realizing what our ancestors have known for thousands of years, that we are all in a perpetual state of vibration, which can be made optimal for healing, regeneration, transformation, and awakenings of all kinds.

So let's get down with the vibrational frequencies...

Ancient Solfeggio Frequencies

Solfeggio Frequencies and their sacred tones were used in ancient Gregorian chants for tremendous spiritual blessings and are said to have great healing power and benefits. This knowledge all but disappeared in about 1000 AD. The tones, with chants sung in Latin, at religious masses, resonated with the subconscious mind to promote great healing and transformation. There were six original sacred tones and three that were recently added based on mathematical progression. Each of these frequencies is believed to have specific purposes.

Solfeggio Frequencies
https://www.youtube.com/results?search_query=Solfeggio

UT – 396 Hz Intent: Turning Grief to Joy, Liberating Guilt and Fear
https://www.youtube.com/results?search_query=Solfeggio+396

This 396 Hz frequency cleanses the feeling for guilt and fear and liberates its energy from your system, including subconscious blockages and negative beliefs.

RE – 417 Hz Intent: Undoing Situations and Facilitating Change
https://www.youtube.com/results?search_query=Solfeggio+417

This 417 Hz frequency brings about inexhaustible sources of energy to bring about change in your life and cleanses destructive influences and traumatic experiences of past events.

MI – 528 Hz Intent: DNA Repair, Cellular Regeneration, Transformation and Miracles
https://www.youtube.com/results?search_query=Solfeggio+528

This 528 Hz frequency brings about transformation and miracles in your life, scientifically proven to have beneficial effects on DNA repair and cellular regeneration, while increasing energy, awareness, creativity, clarity, imagination, intuition, inner peace, celebration and realization of higher purpose.

FA – 639 Hz Intent: Re-connecting and Balancing Relationships
https://www.youtube.com/results?search_query=Solfeggio+639

This 639 Hz frequency brings about harmonious interpersonal relationships with partners, family, friends, and community, while enhancing communication, understanding, tolerance and love.

SOL – 741 Hz Intent: Solutions, Solving Problems and Expressions
https://www.youtube.com/results?search_query=Solfeggio+741

This 741 Hz frequency brings about cleansing of toxins, healthier lifestyle, healthier diet, simpler life, with greater problem solving and self-expression, resulting in a pure and stable life.

LA – 852 Hz Intent: Awakening Intuition and Returning to Spiritual Order
https://www.youtube.com/results?search_query=Solfeggio+852

This 825 Hz frequency brings about intuition with the ability to see through the illusions in your life. It raises awareness allowing you to return to spiritual order. It enables the cells to transform themselves into s system of higher order.

SI – 963 Hz Intent: Awakens any System to its Original Perfect State
https://www.youtube.com/results?search_query=Solfeggio+963

This 963 Hz frequency connects you to light and all-embracing spirit, direct experience, and a return to oneness and true nature.

174 Hz – Intent: Natural Anesthetic
https://www.youtube.com/results?search_query=Solfeggio+174

This 174 Hz frequency reduces physical and emotional pain, promotes a sense of security, safety and love, while helping to reduce stress.

285 Hz – Intent: Return Tissue to its Original Form
https://www.youtube.com/results?search_query=Solfeggio+285

This 295 Hz frequency leaves your body energized and rejuvenated, with improved energy fields and restructure of damaged tissue.

Schumann Resonance Frequency

The Schumann Resonance frequency is found in the ionosphere, one of the layers that makes up the atmosphere, and it is sometimes referred to as the heartbeat of mother earth.

This is the optimum frequency for physical, immune and psychological health, including increased stress tolerance. In ancient times, structures were built to amplify this frequency, to promote healing. In modern society, this frequency is often masked by everyday electronics.

Earth's Vibration – Binaural Beat 7.83 Hz (Schumann Resonance)
https://www.youtube.com/results?search_query=Earth+Schumann+Resonance

Brainwave Frequencies

Alpha Brainwaves range from 8 Hz to 15 Hz and are essential for relaxation and are considered the brain's normal functioning state, or at least it should be, to avoid stress related disease. It is often related to a deeply relaxed state for light meditation and trance.

Highly creative, problem solving, peak performance people tend to spend more time in alpha brainwave states. If that's just not you, the good news is alpha brainwaves can be supplemented to restore balance and creativity.

College students often create their own background mixes of alpha waves during study sessions and it can be the most effective state for mind programming, day dreaming, fantasizing, visualization, and creativity.

Alpha Brainwaves for Creativity, Relaxation and Learning
https://www.youtube.com/results?search_query=alpha+waves

Beta Brainwaves – range between 13 Hz and 40 Hz. many people are stuck with beta waves all day long, from the sense of pressure and stress of getting up in the morning until they finally wind down at the end of the day.

Occupation has a lot to do with this. People, who are forced to do more labor intensive routine tasks that they would not normally do, tend to be stuck in this rut. Caffeine doesn't help matters either; it tends to suppresses alpha and theta brainwaves, so the result is a go-go-go for most people all day long.

This state of mind is generally associated with alertness, active attention, analysis, fast thinking and anxiety, where stresses often take you into the higher ranges.

For people who tend to be more relaxed all the time, but procrastinate, who really need to be wired to cram for a test at school or a project at work, beta brainwaves can be supplemented too.

Beta Brainwaves for Focus, Concentration and Stimulation
https://www.youtube.com/results?search_query=beta+waves

Feel Alive – Beta Brainwave Boost – Isochoric Tones
https://www.youtube.com/results?search_query=Feel+Alive+Beta+Brainwave+Boost

The best balance for alpha brainwaves and beta brainwaves is free flowing alternate states during the day, not locked into a grind, so if necessary, put your iPod mix together and take alpha breaks as needed to rejuvenate.

Delta Brainwaves lower your awareness while you sleep in the ranges of 0.5 Hz to 4 Hz. They are regarded as the most relaxing of the brainwaves, associated with the sub-conscious mind while in a deep dreamless sleep of tranquility. This is the ideal state for the body to heal and rejuvenate.

Delta Brainwave Sleep Meditations
https://www.youtube.com/results?search_query=Delta+Wave+Sleep+Meditations

Thera Brainwaves ranges from 4 Hz to 8 Hz and are often used for REM sleep, super learning, trance, meditation, day dreaming, visualization, creative thinking, tap into inner genius, development of metaphysical abilities, including astral projection, lucid dreaming, and deep spiritual connections.

They have many of the same characteristics as the above brainwave lengths combined, including improved creativity, memory, learning, intuition, energy, healing, inspiration and peak performance, along with better stress tolerances.

There is a huge collection of theta music and meditations available on You Tube.

Chambers of Thought
https://www.youtube.com/results?search_query=chambers+of+thought

Cosmic Traveler
https://www.youtube.com/results?search_query=Cosmic+Traveler

Gateways of Passage
https://www.youtube.com/results?search_query=Gateways+of+Passage

Theta Realms
https://www.youtube.com/results?search_query=Theta+Realms

After listening to theta music, it's good to listen to some alpha brainwaves before getting back to things.

Blue Radiance Alpha Wave Restoration
https://www.youtube.com/results?search_query=Blue+Radiance+Alpha+Restoration

Gamma Brainwaves, not to be confused with gamma rays from a super nova explosion, are very fast, high frequency brainwaves, about 40 Hz and above. They are used for extremely high levels of "In the Zone" cognitive function, concentration, sensory perception, mood, advanced meditation, and conscious elevation.

They are associated with happiness, compassion and feelings of blessings. They are ideal for study, allowing greater focus as you quickly review information, remember it, and retrieve it later. They act as a natural anti-depressant.

Gama Brainwaves – Your Highest Form of Vibration
https://www.youtube.com/results?search_query=Gamma+Waves

Mu Brainwaves are considered a variant of alpha brainwaves that increase during meditation. They are linked to physical activity or watching others while physically activity.

Mu Waves
https://www.youtube.com/results?search_query=mu+waves

Brainwave Entrainment

BWE - Brainwave Entrainment is the process of getting two or more waves to vibrate in harmony.

For centuries people have been using music to induce feelings. BWE takes that to new levels, with benefits that include more energy, better performance, improved relationships and deeper relaxation experiences.

BWE is a proven method to alter your brainwaves for conscious expansion, self-hypnosis and meditation.

Both BWE and listing to individual brainwave frequency ranges will allow you to recognize and experience the various states of consciousness to help you create these states on your own, at will, with practice.

Binaural Beats require a headset. These tones are the most popular brainwave entrainment method. Some benefits include reduced stress, improved concentration, focus, memory, intuition, intelligence, and creativity

The human ear can only hear in the ranges of 20Hz to 20000Hz, so to achieve a frequency lower than 20Hz, in the range of brainwaves, sounds or tones are played in each ear resulting in a third sound or tone resonating in the brain. With his technology, your brainwaves can reach and maintain any frequency you need.

Binaural Beats
https://www.youtube.com/results?search_query=Binaural+Beats

Isochronic Beats are a newer technology that doesn't require headsets. They have the same benefits as binaural beats in a quicker timeframe.

Isochronic Beats
https://www.youtube.com/results?search_query=Isochronic+Beats

Monaural Beats are a newer technology that doesn't require headsets. They use two tones that would be used in binaural beats, but are played in each channel resulting in a stronger stimulus.

Monaural Beats
https://www.youtube.com/results?search_query=Monaural+Beats

Monaural Meditation
https://www.youtube.com/results?search_query=Monaural+Meditation

HemiSync is a trademarked brand for the process used to create audio patterns using binary beats.

Hemisync Meditation
https://www.youtube.com/results?search_query=hemi+sync+meditation

White Noise is a continuum of frequencies distributed equally over the entire hearing range. This is often used as a background noise for studying; relaxation, concentration, focus and to calm the mind.

White Noise
https://www.youtube.com/results?search_query=White+Noise

Classical Music has been shown to enhance mental alertness and memory, improve your sleep quality, relieve your stress levels, reduce depression, manage pain, and promotes openness with yourself and honest communication of ones emotions.

Classical Music
https://www.youtube.com/results?search_query=Classicl+Music

Raising Your Vibrations

Your vibration is a direct reflection of your thoughts, emotions, spoken words, interactions, and actions. Everything in your life impacts your overall personal vibrational threshold, but not all of it is healthy, so it can become necessary to work on it, especially if you are experiencing health problems.

To be vibrant, you need to develop a positive attitude and outlook, trusting that your soul's intention and internal compose will guide you in the right direction, that will serve to build your resilience to stress, while letting go of self-limiting beliefs that tend to hold you back.

Higher vibrational frequencies are associated with empowering thoughts, positive emotions, good health, spiritual awareness, abundance, awakenings and enlightenment. Once you get on this treadmill, it's like a perpetual cycle of personal growth. The higher your vibrational frequency, the more likely you are to attract people and circumstances that are also positive influences, in a "like" attracts "like" sort of way, becoming an ever greater perpetual cycle to ever greater heights in your life.

Operating at higher vibrations of thought is very liberating, with an unbelievable sense of energy and ultimate reality, but the real trick is to get in a mindset where it is sustainable over the long haul. This entire guide is devoted to helping you discover how to achieve consistently higher vibrations, although you may think of it as joy, happiness or peace of mind.

So here are some ideas that can help you raise your vibrations in a very lasting way. Keep in mind that the other sections of this guide will all take you a long way to raising your vibrations, vitality, and health, but here are more tools for your tool belt.

Perhaps the best place to start is to **become more aware of your thoughts**. The next time a negative thought or emotion pops into your heard, acknowledge it, try to turn it into a positive by looking at it from different perspectives, and if necessary, dismiss it by mentally throwing it into a virtual trashcan on the other side of the room.

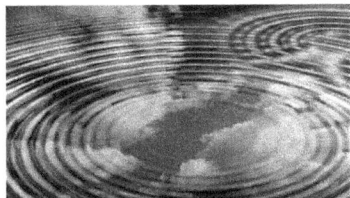 **Drink plenty of water** to help avoid the symptoms of dehydration, help detoxify your system and help keep your energy levels and vibrations high during the day. Even a shower, swim, or Epsom salt bath can be very uplifting, rinsing away your tension.

Individuals holding a cup and even water spoken to or blessed have been shown to have vibration. When this waster is frozen, positive people and expressed words have spectacular snowflake like patterns, while things like heavy metal music resembles something similar to shattered glass.

Your heart muscle, water in your body and movement all serve to carry your vibrations through every fiber of your being, so stay hydrated.

Sign up for some **positive quotes of the day** to serve as a reminder of your desire to raise your vibrations and develop more of a vibrant personality.

Allow your spiritual roots to penetrate every fiber of your being and your entire life. Try taking small steps towards your soul's purpose, or find a good mentor to help you discover what that purpose is.

Volunteer your time to worthy causes that will help make you happier, personally fulfilled and healthier.

Find things in your life, or around you, to appreciate and be grateful. Take a moment each day to reflect on those things more. Simply taking a moment to look around at a view can do wonders for your vibrations.

Practice simple or even random acts of kindness without expecting anything in return. If you go through a car pool to work each day, try paying for the car behind you. You might be surprised at the reaction of the person in that car along with the toll both operator.

Spend time with high vibrational friends and visit places that are of high vibrations, such as concerts.

Choose one exercise that you enjoy and slip it into your daily routine. Aside from keeping you fit, this will help to keep your vibrational energies flowing. Even 10 minutes a day will work wonders.

Spend more time doing activities that you enjoy, find inspiring or are passionate about each day; like yoga, getting back to nature, taking a trip to the lake or ocean.

Spend more time smiling and laughing, with friends, family or even with the selection of TV shows you choose to tune into, or just get out to a comedy club every now and then.

Sing and dance more, even if it's just a dance for one in your room or bathroom. Try getting out to some karaoke, even if you need to get out of your comfort zone to do it.

Organize Your Environment because your emotional state often mirrors your physical environment, so the simple act of doing chores can be an instant energy boost.

Let go of the need for perfection. The path to higher awareness is not linear, perfection is always a moving target because your perception is always evolving, Simply put, if it's worth doing, it's worth moving on it now rather than waiting for perfection. Simply take an iterative, agile or one step after another approach to getting things done.

Pursue remarkable new adventures. To be truly happy, you must experience that feeling and allow it to resonate and persist through you.

Take Action and Claim Responsibility. It's always easier to apologize afterwards than to ask for permission. Even if it's only small steps, take charge of your situation, set goals for yourself and your personal growth, focus on your desires and soul's intention and above all, take action!

Take a step outside of your comfort zone and face your fears. to expose greater opportunities and possibilities.

Simply let go of your baggage and other peoples baggage too, let go of the past, clear out the cobwebs, and allow yourself to live in the moment, with a happy and fulfilling life.

Simply let go with forgiveness once boundaries have been re-established and agreed upon.

Allow your true self to vibrate brightest of all. Like an actor, we all put on masks for the occasion to play the part, but let your true self shine the brightest of all. Choose the path of most resistance when the opportunity presents itself to transform your life in new ways.

Open yourself to love for yourself and others with compassion and empathy. Even when life throws you a curve ball, keep your composure, stay patient with yourself, remember life is about growing so mistakes are going to happen, and turn it into a win rather than getting down on yourself.

Put gossip and negativity in the waste basket. Ultimately, gossip, negativity, and complaining will bring your vibrational energy levels down.

Personal growth is all about self-discovery, so spend time learning, reading, writing and understanding to raise your vibrations and guide your transformation.

Strive for balance. You don't need to overdo it just to achieve a more vibrant way of life, simply take steps in the right direction. If you are trying to restore your wellbeing, take some bigger steps.

Take up some of the tips throughout this book, especially the breathing exercises, meditation and stress relief ones.

Listen to ancient Buddhist and Gregorian chants to shift your frequency.

Take a look at NLP - Neuro-Linguistic Programing Training, involving the three most influential components involved in producing human experience: neurology, language and programming.

https://www.youtube.com/results?search_query=NLP

Transcend limitation and obtain your wildest dreams by understanding the power of your thoughts, feelings, and spoken words and taking control of those elements within you.

Allow yourself some "me" time, in a place that is peaceful and would allow you to reflect, meditate, or express yourself in vibrant ways.

Low Frequency Vibrations are Energy Vampires

Viral Energy Influences

The other day I heard on the radio that Americans are sick or don't feel up to par about 142 days of the year, that's almost 40% of the time or an astonishing 3 days a week. Vitamin D reduces your chances of getting the flu and vitamin C reduces the duration of colds, but there are a lot of things out there that can get the best of you.

Although each section in this guide could be used separately or in unison to help you overcome your challenges, this section specifically covers chronic fatigue, disease, conditions, cancer, tumors, and viruses.

According to the CDC - Centers for Disease Control, CFS - Chronic Fatigue Syndrome "is a debilitating and complex disorder characterized by profound fatigue that is not improved by bed rest and that may be worsened by physical or mental activity. Symptoms affect several body systems and may include weakness, muscle pain, impaired memory and/or mental concentration, and insomnia, which can result in reduced participation in daily activities".

According to the CDC, EBV - Epstein - Barr virus "is one of the most common human viruses in the world. It spreads primarily through saliva. EBV can cause infectious mononucleosis, also called mono, and other illnesses. Most people will get infected with EBV in their lifetime and will not have any symptoms. Mono caused by EBV is most common among teens and adults.

Although EBV accounts for 90% of all mononucleosis cases, its cousin CMV – Cytomegalovirus accounts for the other 10% of the cases. Both of these viruses can lay dormant for years and cause crippling long lasting fatigue.

According to the CDC, "CMV is a common virus that infects people of all ages. Most CMV infections are "silent," meaning most people who are infected with CMV have no signs or symptoms. However, CMV can cause disease in people with a weakened immune system and in babies infected before birth. About 1 in 150 children are born with congenital (present at birth) CMV infection."

Overall, about 99% of the population is infected with at least one or more viruses in this particular family of viruses, which goes beyond epidemic proportions, never mind all the other pathogens we are exposed to on a daily bases.

Over 30 years ago I was working at an old PVC/Polyco manufacturing plant in the former "Plastics Capital of the World". I was actually there to help shut down the facility and bring up operations at two new locations in different parts of the county.

It was the first gorgeous spring day and I was extremely inspired to open my office window. Little did I know that this one single act would change my life forever?

Just as the window opened, a gust of wind blew dust from the window sill into my face. By the next morning, many lymph nodes under my chin and on my neck were extremely enlarged, accompanied by extreme fatigue.

The condition spread like a cancer, the fatigue was like an infection, yet it was obviously the result of exposure to a hazardous environment material.

Keeping this condition in check was an ongoing battle for over 20 years. Although I learned many techniques to resolve inflamed lymph nodes, it resulted in nine surgeries, because I couldn't beat the lymph nodes that had the dust in them. Often the surgeries made the medical journals because of the size of the lymph nodes, the initial pathologies almost always suggested cancer, yet I was always sent home with not so much as a hint on how to manage the condition for myself.

Many doctors have argued with my methods to manage the condition, but not one of them has had anything constructive to add as a course of treatment. I've followed cancer research and virus research for years, along with general health research, so it wasn't difficult to justify my approach in terms they could relate with.

It all started out rather simple and progressed from there:

- Large amounts of caffeinated coffee to keep my body borderline dehydrated and slow down the progression of the decease.
- Smoking to compensate for all the coffee, while helping to reduce stress and allow me to focus on my particular line of work, which requires a lot of creativity.
- Low to Moderate Exercise only – lymph nodes are like small pumps that rely on exercise to keep them flowing, again to slow down the progression of the disease.
- Good Nutrition, Stress Management and Meditation– see the Physical Energies section of this guide.
- Homemade Juices - See the Energizer drink below.
- Numerous Supplements, Homeopathic Remedies, Over the Counter Drugs, Allergy Medications, and Pharmaceuticals, all with more of a trial and failure style approach, mostly with mixed results.

My only real advantage with this condition was it progressed slowly, allowing me plenty of time to experiment. I had some idea what the cause actually was and had a basic understanding of how the progression was occurring, which is more than most people get with chronic conditions, syndromes, or diseases.

My first major breakthrough was a homemade juice that I affectionately called the "Energizer". It had one bunch of Parsley, a couple Apples and topped off with Carrots. This solved the fatigue problem, but it wasn't until I finally beat the EBV virus that I understood why...

The Parsley in the juice leaves a zinc or metallic aftertaste, which is perhaps the simplest and only way to tell if you have an active EBV infection. It does much more than that though, there is something in the Parsley that binds to the virus and temporarily renders it inert.

My next major breakthrough was coming across some virus research that showed the EBV virus hyper reacts to plasticizers, a substance used to make plastics soft and pliable. That is exactly what I was observing and confirmed EBV as my primary suspect and culprit involved in the progression of the disease. I would never again drink from cheap or flimsy plastic bottles that could leach chemicals into the beverage, especially when it sits on a hot truck or in the back of a store before refrigeration.

My next major breakthrough was trying Prednisone before a surgery. Within several days the pain was too great to take, so went I with my first thought, an Energizer juice with the Apples substituted for Beats, followed by a shot of Nyquil as a chaser. This made me extremely thirsty, drinking water frequently. I called the effect "Super Hydration", which was more than enough to overpower the Prednisone for a couple of days. Once the pain returned, I simply repeated the juice. After my third juice, numerous inflamed lymph nodes literally exploded. I had a beer to celebrate.

The effect of Super Hydration was really interesting, stretching out ells in a way where it would be hard to believe any unhealthy cells could survive. Beet juice on its own is known to have miraculous effects at taking out tumors. There is some risk; I learned later it is possible to drown cells under the right circumstances. Also, you can't eat sold foods while doing this. I made the mistake of eating one spoonful of cereal and got thousands of lacerations in my mouth. I also had a good size piece of chicken go down the wrong way in a one way valve under my lounge.

The Prednisone nailed the EBV virus, crushing it like the bug. There were two pockets of the virus in my tongue that were very painful to eliminate. It also stripped away the viral shedding in my throat. I did some research on Prednisone afterwards and there were some articles suggesting it was effective against the EBV virus, but it didn't sound like that was accepted by mainstream medicine yet, probably because they don't have a way to check for and active EBV infection. Now you do, with the Energizer juice.

As I understand EBV at this point, it just reduces the severity of other infections, especially in the throat, but increases the duration. It has many ways to trick your immune system into thinking it is something else like a bacteria, so when it gets involved, it generally gets in the way,

For example with Cancer, you want your immune system on task, not side tracked by something like EBV, so it is good to get this virus under control. I mainly became interested in cancer research because of all the X-Rays and CAT scans, sometimes effecting blemishes on my skin, but more so because that was always the biggest concern with all of my surgeries.

The underlying cause of cancer is always radiation from the sun, cosmic rays, nuclear testing, or naturally occurring radioactive isotopes that breaks down the DNA in cells. Next, you need a catalyst, such as a carcinogen or virus or bacteria known to cause abnormal cell growth. Finally, you need a weekend immune system, because everyone gets some cancer cells and under normal circumstances your body can easily deal with them. So the same thing you need to do for prevention works for remission, which is simply to get healthy and improve the immune response as you go through surgery and chemotherapy treatment.

The battle wasn't over... There was still one isolated lymph node that was spreading to adjacent nodes. I wanted to get it with the Prednisone and Super Hydration, but the chicken down the wrong pipe was a big distraction involving an emergency room visit. In time I realized I had the perfect circumstances to figure out what was going on here.

I found a homeopathic allergy remedy that you dissolve under tongue. After taking it at a much higher dosage than recommended for about a week, the lymph nodes shrank and back flushed into the blood stream, resulting in a short-term mononucleosis, which has such a distinct feeling to it, that it can't be mistaken for anything else.

The amazing thing about this is if you stop the allergy treatment too soon, the virus will once again return to the infected lymph nodes in the exact same proportions as before. Continue the allergy treatment longer, the immune system can easily deal with the virus in the blood stream and the lymph nodes returned to normal size. This was proof that there was something else involved that EBV was attracted to and hyper reacting to.

Not being able to learn anything more from this last large lymph node, I finally got it removed. The oncologist that I talked to afterwards thought the only way I could have exploded lymph nodes with Prednisone was if there was a yeast or fungus involved in the infection. Since I spent some time in the Ohio region, the prudent thing to do was get checked for Histoplasma, but that was negative just like every other test.

That gave me a great idea though... I got some magnesium oxide and let a table spoon full dissolve under my tongue. Sure enough, there was a fungal infection in my front saliva gland on the left side. Exposing it in this manner was all it took for my immune system to do the rest.

This was the cause of the progressive infection, but I still cannot put a name to it, along with its copartner EBV. Even so, both were eradicated. I haven't seen either since. Even my Energizer juice lost its aftertaste, zing and appeal, so I rarely drink that anymore.

That left one remaining lymph node in my chest that was inoperable. I've suspected for some time that this lymph node was different, leaching into my system, causing a peripheral neuropathy in my feet. My oncologists mentioned that a number of his cancer patients had that problem.

My plan was simple, hydration, exercise and mind-body stimulation to take out this node. It worked all too well, to the point where I was doing the mind-body stimulations in my sleep.

When the node went, it was like a bomb went off in my body. It work me suddenly with sever heart palpitations. Some of this went directly into the bloodstream; the rest went mostly to my hands. I soaked my hands in vinegar and took Benadryl to help save the nerves. In time, I managed to spread this out over my entire body, causing a systemic peripheral neuropathy. I saw a dermatologist because of the many types of blemishes and rashes that developed. It was all just common floras, the kind of thing he sees every day, but none of it was usual for me.

I sensed the VZV - Varicelle Zoster Virus involvement, yet another cousin of EBV and CMV. According to the CDC, this virus is responsible for Chickenpox and Shingles, but they don't even begin to cover the research I've seen. This virus goes dormant in the nerves and years later when the virus reactivates if causes a wide range of diseases and neurological conditions even in individuals with an otherwise healthy immune response. This is one nasty virus that also gets involved with everything.

For years I wanted a full body assault on this problem rather than dealing with one lymph node at a time. Now I had my change. I stuck with the hydration, exercise and mind-body approach, but tried various allergy medications too. Nothing seemed to work, this had to be just another overgrowth of flora, but it was resilient and hard to beat.

VZV is treatable using acyclovir for chickenpox, valaciclovir for the shingles, zoster-immune globulin (ZIG) and vidarabine VZV immune globulin. The CDC recommends two doses of chickenpox vaccine for children, adolescents, and adults.

Instead of resorting to medication specific to the virus, I really wanted to take it out myself. Finally, once I learned how to raise my vibrations, my entirely mind over matter approach worked almost effortlessly. I'm not sure how much of the virus I actually got, but the peripheral neuropathy is gone.

We will be getting into high vibrational approaches in the next chapter.

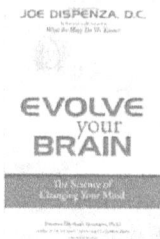

Dr. Joe Dispenza, author of Evolve Your Brain: The Science of Changing Your Mind claims that through neuroplasticity, a person can rewire their brain. In his research, he discovered that those who had achieved total healing from terminal disease were able to rewire their brain through positive intention and thought. He explains thoughts create chemical reactions that keep you addicted to patterns and feelings, so by breaking these patterns, it's possible to evolve/reprogram your brain.

Pathogens and Chemicals are Energy Vampires

Chapter II – The Metaphysical Experience

Awakenings of All Kinds Can Change Your Life

Awakenings generally refer to a form of Eastern spiritual enlightenment and the realization there is more to the universe and reality, beyond the "3rd dimension".

Your perspective on life is constantly changing, but awakenings can often happen spontaneously, so how you spend your time can change dramatically.

The Meaning of Life is a Jigsaw Puzzle

In my younger days, things were much simpler. Just tried to live life to the fullest, live in the moment, make the most of it as if it was my last day, with as many rich experiences as possible, with a great career, lifestyle, family life, etc. and a few bumps along the way!

Midlife I had a few health related issues that took years to overcome, mostly from trial and error, and largely from following my inspirations and ideas.

Life's Ultimate Truth and Purpose of Life

Later in life, I personally had two spiritual awakenings, among many other types of awakenings. One of these was a Shaman Calling, followed by my True Calling a year later. If you believe in evolving and gaining experience, which some believe happens over many lifetimes, this could happen to you anytime.

My Shaman calling was rather intense, while my true calling was rather dramatic, which was the simplest aspect about the universe that I'm supposed to focus on for some reason, which is that we live in a duality on 4-d space-time. So now I research and write papers for science journals; although I thought my homework days were long behind me.

I'm somewhat of a skeptical traveler when it comes to reading about spiritual matters that others have experienced, but here I was in complete amazement.

If you have an interest, read about Tesla, the inventor of electricity, he had stories to tell that makes my homework assignment look trivial.

After doing much research, I learned this wasn't that uncommon, and in many ways resembles inspiration. Some awakenings are gradual with signs, others are dramatic and spontaneous, but many types and levels of awakenings are achievable by anybody, shifting between states or levels of consciousness, using a wide range of techniques and traditions to achieve.

Signs of Gradual Awakenings

- Realizing you have a stronger connection with nature, the earth, or the universe
- Realizing you have a strong interest in health, diet, physical fitness, or taking care of yourself
- Realizing there is a deeper meaning waiting to be discovered
- Realizing your sleeping patterns are changing, with periods of intense energy
- Realizing you have a thirst for personal growth, esoteric knowledge, the new age movement, or other religions or societies
- Realizing that you have less interest in material things
- Realizing that you have less in common with old friends
- Realizing you are more interested in the pursuit of knowledge and wisdom
- Realizing you have a desire to reconnect with your higher self
- Realizing that your belief system is evolving
- Realizing your mind, body, soul are ready to transform
- Realizing you could help make the world a better place
- Realizing there is more to life
- Realizing you no longer fear death
- Realizing that you are a spiritual being that is timeless and eternal, learning how to live a physical existence.
- Realizing that coincidences keep appearing in your life, synchronicity
- Realizing your calling, deepest desires and passions are surfacing
- Realizing you have a deeper feeling of bliss towards life
- Realizing you have received a Shamanic calling
- Realizing you have glimpses of the cosmic consciousness
- Realizing you relate to prana and cosmic energy more and more

The Challenges of Everyday Life

In short, moving things along quicker often involves simply following your inspirations first and foremost, but if you are good with more of a scenic route, explore your interests, passions, desires, dreams, etc. too.

The Quest for Enlightenment is More Challenging

Enlightenment can mean different things to different people, such as being enlightened, or the Age of Enlightenment, which was an intellectual and philosophical movement. Often it is referred to as a higher state of consciousness or plain of existence.

Spiritual Enlightenment often has its roots in several religions including, Hinduism (moksha and mukti), Buddhism (bodhi, kensho and satoru), Jainism (jnana) and Zoroastrianism (ushta).

Although yoga (India origins) appears to focus on controlling the body, it is an ancient spiritual discipline, a form of meditation, harnessing breathing techniques (pranayama) and the energy of the body (prana) to tame the mind and passions, with attentions to various states of consciousness and forms of trance states that can be achieved by focusing on a single object or thought, such as a word or candle flame, to achieve liberation (moksha and mukti) and perfection (poorna).

The Buddha strives to achieve serenity, compassion, generosity, wisdom, enlightenment, and spirituality to transcend the limitations of the body and break the cycle of karma and endless reincarnation. The Buddha taught meditation as a transformative practice to relax heart and wake to the moment, involving the body and mind as a single entity. Some methods involve reflection on life's lessons, often in trance like states, to obtain the supreme and ultimate awareness and wisdom of the universe, surrendering to nirvana, bliss, and awakenings that already exist within you.

Although there is many differences, the similarities include an end to suffering, persistence (no going back) and transcendence, often involving forms of meditation that calm the mind to achieve.

Unless someone is trying to recruit you into some religious group, or charging you for assistance of some kind, most will tell you the odds are not in your favor to achieve more than seeking enlightenment with perhaps some expansion of consciousness's along the way.

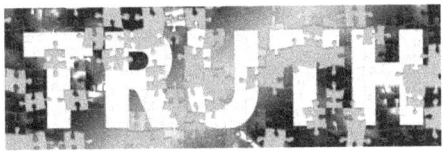

As Ginsa Charles put it, "The degree to which your Consciousness expands, is the degree to which you understand yourself and the universe."

How to Reach Your Minds Potential

The brain weighs 3 pounds, uses 20% of the energy demands of the body.

Any given snapshot of the brain shows between 10–15% of the brain being active, a stimulating conversion over 10 minutes results in about 40% of the brain being active, while as much as 100% of the brain is active over a 24 hour period.

Even so, there is a lot of merit in using more of the brain at once, or even more of the trillions of neuroconnectors at once.

Striving to excel is always great on so many levels, but its hard to say exactly how far any of us will eventually be able to grow as a species.

There are probably so many things that have influenced our evolution over many millennia. The fossil record suggests that we have been evolving quicker over the last five thousand years by as much as seven percent.

Scientists have suggested as we solve more problems, such as microbes and viruses, we will have less reason to evolve in the future, so we may need to take charge of our own evolution at some point.

Right now the only control we have over self-evolving is through life's experiences, and even though it is more of a biological function to pass on good genes, it also serves to actuate genes.

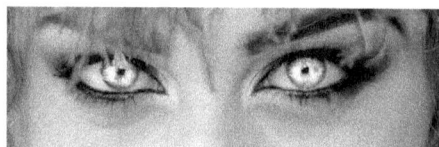

What are the Chances of Becoming Enlightened?

Enlightenment can mean different things to different people, such as the state of being enlightened, or even the Age of Enlightenment, which was an intellectual and philosophical movement. Enlightenment can often mean much more than any of that, taking it all too new heights, achieving a higher plain of existence, with more than one path to follow.

The Dual Paths to Enlightenment

Our ancestors were much more in tune with nature, probably with a deeper and more profound belief system, not just going through the motions, which would have been a huge benefit in achieving enlightenment.

Alexander the Great's vast empire opened the door to Eastern religion and mysticism to the west, while Greek philosophy and reason moved east starting around 340BC. This vast mixing of various religious and philosophical ideas has continued through the centuries, despite attempts from organized religion to suppress it, to reach a global scale and the dawn of a new age.

To become truly enlightened, you need to be self-reliant, have a passion for personal growth, constantly seeking knowledge and wisdom, be fearless of the unknown, have a spirit for adventure, enjoy the journey, demonstrate perseverance to stay the path, be good under pressure, rationalize over the many mysteries discovered, learn how your own mind-body really works, and even learn how to defend yourself on many levels.

This is not exactly a typical curriculum, you're setting out on your own path, at your own pace with your faith and some good online resources to help you get started, such as this book and many disciplines and traditions, such as yoga, pranayama, prana, cosmic energy, tie chi, Zen, and meditation, etc.

Your first significant milestone is duality, and this isn't entirely just a spiritual journey, it will bring you much closer to nature and the universe too. You're going to need to explore duality, before reaching its plateau of enlightenment and moving beyond, which I'm starting to believe is exponential. This of course assumes you are going to master reality somewhere along the way as well.

Your awareness of greater aspects to reality and duality can happen gradually or spontaneously, often with many inspirations and awakenings to guide you, but you may need to handle new situations without freaking out too.

It's much more than just reading about opening your third-eye or raising your kundalini, or even being aware of such things, and there is no going back either.

The journey through reality and eventually duality will greatly expand your consciousness along the way. In short, this venture can be described as pealing an onion, just to discover there is yet more to it all, and again there is no going back! Many will tell you the odds are not in your favor.

This can be an exciting journey, but a somewhat reckless way to go, just diving right in, with risks that are high and so are the rewards, which is the path I took, or should I say was chosen for me, with some hard lessons learned along the way, but there is another more gradual way that involves finding life's ultimate truth.

The gradual approach simply involves following your inspirations, interests, passions, desires and goals, not in any particular order, but if you are in more of a hurry to reach enlightenment, follow your inspirations foremost. This is more along the lines of the scenic route, to learn life's lessons and skills that you will need for your journey, but some meditation for self-reflection can help move thing along.

We may never fully comprehend everything about reality, but healthcare will always be mediocre at best, until we scientifically recognize there is more to reality than most people can perceive, that can influence our health, energy, well-being, stress levels and state of mind in both good and adverse ways; Shakti research will ultimately reveal a duality that will greatly impact healthcare.

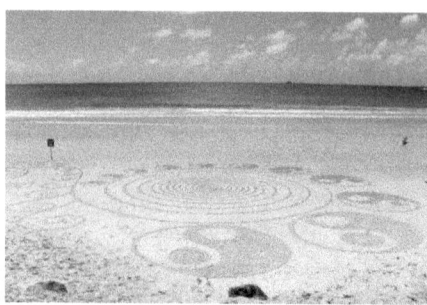

Where Does the Rabbit Hole Go and How Deep Is It?

Many of us seek the truth about our origins, spirituality, purpose and the nature of reality in our own way. Some take the scenic route, one step at a time, thought by many to take place over many lifespans, while others take the road less traveled.

As your understanding of nature and the universe expands, its abundantly clear that reality is more amazing than fiction, that life and nature is more prevalent than most could possibly conceive, that there has to be more to life after this reality, and the entire journey is an odyssey of the mind like no other, with all kinds of challenges along the way.

As much as it seems like this journey is going somewhere specific, and it might be, we may not even be capable of conceiving how deep the rabbit hole goes.

There is a lot of insight about the rabbit hole that can be read on the web and in and throughout this book that can help as a guide without being so much of a spoiler, including Prana, Shakti, Kundalini, Third-Eye, Synchronicity and Spiritual awakenings.

You will hear many similarities about the path to enlightenment too, such as overcoming ego and suffering and achieving persistence, but everyone has their own challenges to overcome with what could be a very different journey.

So all I can really say is enjoy all the wonders and enjoy the ride!

The State of "Persistent" Enlightenment Explained

Enlightenment has different meanings in many cultures and religions, including spiritual enlightenment and intellectual enlightenment.

There are also multiple paths, including duality and non-duality, with similar beliefs and religions including Hinduism and Buddhism, with variations on nirvana and things like karma and reincarnation.

Because of all these cultural and religious differences, and because awakenings often happen spontaneously without a clear understanding by the person experiencing them, there is difficulty getting a common consensus in regards to enlightenment.

Enlightenment can take many years and depending on the path you take could involve numerous awakenings including Prana, Shakti, Kundalini, Third-Eye, Synchronicity and finally Spiritual. There is a non-duality path that doesn't necessarily involve as many awakenings, whereas the duality path goes through everything and gets you experience for a "persistent" enlightenment.

Spiritual Awakenings are very memorable.

Intellectual enlightenment is also high energy and your body seems to produce a Shakti of its own for this. Spiritual Enlightenment seems to be the same thing with a profound bliss and/or love in the mix. For any of this to be "persistent", you need a healthy physical and subtle body, overcome ego, overcome desire, and overcome suffering. The word "overcome" is probably misnomer, because taming ego takes some effort, but lack of desire or suffering is much more natural and just happens after your Spiritual Awakening.

Since enlightenment involves "Shakti", you need to learn from friends, sparing partners, whatever to get good at defending yourself for a consistent and persistent enlightenment.

Enlightenment does not mean all knowing, but it certainly opens your eyes in many ways, with a very clear and fast thought process.

As a kid, everything is wonderment, but as you grow and learn, some of this wonder is greatly diminished or replaced by knowledge and more wonders. Awakenings can also have that effect, with new found perceptions on the world.

Each awakening in your life brings you that much closer to understanding and even getting a better vantage or taste of what enlightenment is all about.

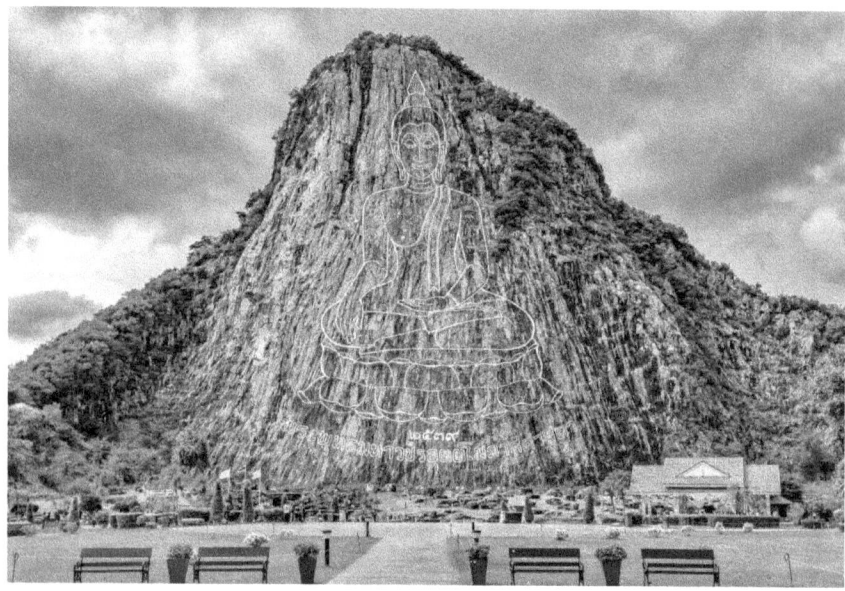

How Scientific is Kundalini Third-Eye Awakenings?

Third-Eye Scientific Proofs

In 1886, two independent anatomists found that the pineal gland was an eye. Subsequent research proves the gland responds to light, similar to your physical eyes, with a melatonin level influence from light, which helps to moderate sleep.

http://www.vivo.colostate.edu/hbooks/pathphys/endocrine/otherendo/pineal.html

Further research suggests the pineal gland determines when sexual awakening begins in children, along with ongoing sexual development. It also produces DMT predominately in children, which decreases during puberty as the pituitary gland becomes more prominent.

Part of what many call a spiritual awakening is to return to this child like state.

The gland also serves as a reservoir for the hormone serotonin, a precursor to melatonin, which suggests the gland is responsible for regulating the chemistry of altered states of consciousness, and the gland probably serves multiple purposes, so scientific findings are far from conclusive.

http://www.wakingtimes.com/2013/04/09/mysteries-of-the-pineal-gland/

There are many current and ancient cultures that regarded this gland as the third-eye, some dating back as far as 13 century BC.

http://www.wakingtimes.com/2016/04/11/mysteries-pineal-gland-ignored-mainstream-science-research/

In recent years, there has been greater interest in uncovering the remaining mysteries of the pineal gland, with at least 10 international conferences that have been devoted to finding its secretes.

Shakti Scientific Proofs

Democritus, a Greek philosopher from the 5th century BC, came up with the first quantum theory describing "atomos", as he called atoms, which were specific to the material that they composed, could have collisions, rebound or stick together, so dissociation's or combinations of these atoms could result in changes in matter.

Shakti goes back as much as the 17th century BC in the written record, but who knows how far back mankind has recognized this primal and essential energy of the universe for health, vitality and longevity.

The substantial evidence is in the various cultures and terms used to explain it, including Hindu Shakti, Prana, Apana and Yyana, Chinese Chi (Qi), Vietnamese Khi, Korean Gi, Japanese Ki, subtle energy and woo energy, Hebrew koach-ha-guf, Greek Bios, English Aether, Cosmic Energy, and Kundalini Energy, American Indians Orenda, Polynesian Mana, and Ancient Germans Od, and Scientifically known as Dark Matter which are believed to be a part of any living thing, translating to breath, air, gas, or life force that permeates the universe.

Cosmic energy (Shakti vapors) is essential to life, yet the closest thing we have to a scientific declaration of its existence is Dark Matter, which isn't even close to being fully understood.

https://universalduality.quora.com/

This is also based on dark matter candidates coming out of UC Irvine, which often resembles similar halo profiles as cold dark matter (CDM), but solves larger than predicted elastic cross section problems, which could be the right size if dark matter is composite. For more information see:

http://www.amazon.com/dp/1520306318

Once you have opened your third-eye correctly, it will open your eyes to a duality with Shakti, entirely new levels of social interactions, and greater awareness.

What if I told you this duality had considerable and even exotic wildlife that many can sense to some extent or another? Would you believe it could have significant influence on your health, wellbeing and energy levels? How would you really know it exists without experiencing it for yourself?

There are scientifically proven things like neutrinos and various forms of energy that we can't see under normal circumstances too, but that's not as interesting as discovering life right under our noises in what could be called a pseudo parallel universe, although it's hard to say how soon further scientific advancements will occur related to particles beyond our normal visual perspective.

Ultimately, the only real proof is in experiencing it for yourself. I could write volumes on the topic and still not cover everything. Besides, although most share similar experiences, when it comes to spiritual awakenings in particular, it is more of a personal journey and vision quest.

Chakra Scientific Proofs

Chakras are even more subjective, as part of the subtle body, which isn't understood by science, except to say Dark Matter/Shakti is being researched and again progress is extremely slow.

From personal experience I can tell you that I was on my journey for about four years before realizing chakras are real. I thought it was just a meditation tool, but you can actually find them once you are awake. They don't really need to be cleansed though, that part is just a tool for meditating. They are coil like focal points on the lining of your subtle body that can be used to ignite Shakti.

In yogic tradition, there are only 7 significant chakras. In actually, there are only 7 chakras period, and any part of the lining can be ignited too, which is easier to think of than countless chakras throughout your body.

They are not as mysterious as they might appear once you have awaken, and the only one you really need to worry about for your first awakening is the root chakra and kundalini.

Kundalini Scientific Proofs

Your kundalini is simply a tornado like force that rises from your root chakra. It changes the rhythm of your body in a positive way that people can sense and tend to be drawn to, but its main purpose is to vaporize prana/Shakti for your brain. As far as science is concerned your brain demands only 20% of the energy consumed from diet, but it is actually much higher than that when you consider prana/cosmic energy, so this gives you a real energy boost, both mentally and physically and will certainly put you in the zone.

Western medical science appears to be ignoring this one. There is such a thing as an overactive Kundalini, aka kundalini syndrome. It is so obvious what the problem is that anybody could make the diagnosis. Doctors must see patients with this condition regularly, but it's hard to say how often anybody gets a prescribed treatment, or even a straight answer about what the problem is, and may even need to endure this condition for years before figuring out how simple it is to resolve.

There lies the problem with trying to become all you can be, to gain greater awareness about reality in general, to experience greater awakenings like synchronicity, to become spiritually awakened or even strive for enlightenment for that matter. There is a lot of incomplete and misinformation out there, and you are proceeding without a safety net, so you can experience many challenges, problems and obstacles that you can't necessarily predict or count on professional help for.

There are probably good reasons why we are being sheltered from the unknown, with things like fluoride, lack of interest in meta-science, and mediocre healthcare at best. It's largely because they know more than they are saying, but not enough to have better options or treatments for that matter, so they are sticking their proverbial heads in the ground, with very slow scientific headway, often just winging it with patient care.

Awakenings are a real eye opener on so many levels. You really need to be ready for it and be able to handle everything that happens, which takes years, or even the rest of your life, depending on how you go about it. Follow the links on this answer to get a better idea if any of this is right for you at this time.

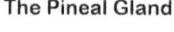

The Pineal Gland

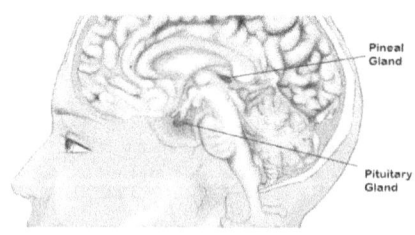

Mind Subtle Body Activation Primers and Prerequisites

The Pineal Gland "Third-Eye" Decalcification

The Pineal Gland, sometimes referred to as the mind's eye or third eye, has been a mystery to mankind for centuries, often thought to be an obsolete remnant of evolution. In recent years, scientists have been more interested in unraveling its mysteries.

In 1880's, two independent teams of anatomists found that the pineal gland was an eye. Subsequent research proves the gland responds to light, similar to your physical eyes. This has been the belief of Indian traditions for centuries, the 'third-eye'. Further research suggests the pineal gland determines when sexual awakening begins in children. The gland also serves as a reservoir for the hormone serotonin, a precursor to melatonin, suggesting the gland is responsible for regulating the chemistry of altered states of consciousness.

The pineal gland is shaped like a pea sized pine-cone, located at the top of the spinal cord within the brain, which is basically a mirror image of the right and left hemisphere except for the pineal gland and the pituitary gland, considered to be the highest control over the endocrine system.

Several years ago I started having an interest in awakening the pineal gland for higher awareness, intuition and experience. This was essentially to free my consciousness from its everyday state. This gland has not been fully functioning since I was a kid. I searched for an answer to this and found that calcification of the gland was the likely culprit, with a couple of possible causes.

The easiest thing to check for is vitamin D deficiency. The parathyroid gland which regulates vitamin D is not particularly smart. It draws both vitamin D and calcium at the same time, so if vitamin D is deficient, it will keep trying, so excessive calcium is continuously drawn from the bones, which acts as a reservoir for calcium. This excessive calcium needs to be excreted or reabsorbed, but most people's intake of calcium is often too high to begin with, so calcium starts building up in soft tissue resulting in hardening, calcification, many diseases and ultimately even death.

Many people also blame fluoride as the cause of calcification of the pineal gland. This halides family of elements which also includes chlorine and bromide, often found in drinking water, binds to Iodine receptors, resulting in iodine deficiency which can cause hypothyroidism, weakling of the immune function, thyroid enlargement, and eventually mental imbalance, mental retardation, brain damage, and autism, all with serious symptoms.

How to Decalcify Your Pineal Gland by Erin Janus
https://www.youtube.com/results?search_query=How+to+Decalcify+Your+Pineal+Gland+by+Erin+Janus

How to Activate and Open Your Third Eye by Teal Swan
https://www.youtube.com/results?search_query=Activate+Open+Your+Third+Eye+Teal+Swan

Nascent Iodine allows the body to cleanse sodium fluoride from the body through the urine as calcium fluoride. Even one dose of iodine almost doubles this excretion of calcium fluoride. It supports the thyroid, which is essential for the pineal gland detoxification, normal hormone balance and endocrine function. This halogen family of elements, including fluoride, chlorine and bromine, lodges itself in iodine receptors, causing iodine deficiency, which can result in hypothyroidism, weakling of the immune function, thyroid enlargement, and ultimately more severe diseases and symptoms. Having enough Iodine available is essential for detoxification of the pineal gland. It also aids with regulating blood sugar, improves brain function, improves metabolism, reduces anxiety, improves thyroid function, and supports normal immune function.

Foods rich in Iodine include bananas, cranberries, dark leafy green vegetables, green beans, kale, kelp, lobster, seaweed and shrimp. Too much Iodine can be toxic to the body, so it is important to consume it regularly, but not overdo it.

Skate Liver Fish Oil with Activator X (Vitamin K1/K12) allows the body to cleanse calcium deposits from various locations, including the pineal gland. This Omega 3 with DHA has been proven to renew neurological brain functions, with remarkable increases in energy. It regulates calcium distribution, which helps with atherosclerosis, osteoporosis, and tooth decay. Vitamin K1 (phyloquinone) is also found in leafy vegetables. Vitamin K2 (menaquinones) is also obtained from intestinal flora, liver, egg yolks, cheese, butter, marine oils, fish eggs and shellfish.

Selenium is a natural way to neutralize sodium fluoride in your body. It can be supplemented at 200mg daily and a rich source is Brazil nuts, which is about 70mg of Selenium per serving. The upper limit of Selenium set by the National Institute of health is 400mg. It is essential for cognitive function and healthy immune function.

Boron is an important trace mineral that can cleanse the body of fluoride. It is also available in beets and dried plums, or in the form of Borax, which is an inexpensive supplement. It should be taken in small amounts during the day, perhaps mixed with water with as little as 1/8 a teaspoon of borax per liter. Another alternative is food grade Sodium Borate. It helps with aging, allergies, arthritis, candida albicans, lupus erythematosus, parasites, osteoporosis, menopause, and sex hormones.

Magnesium Bicarbonate can be added to drinking water to decalcify the pineal gland, alkalize your body, eliminate calcium deposits in your body and significantly increase life expediency. Magnesium is a mineral that is essential to body function. Bicarbonate is a mineral that transports oxygen in the body and buffers acidity. Together they can help with numerous diseases, including arthritis, atherosclerosis, brain calcification, fibromyalgia, gallstones, heart palpitations and liver calcification.

Oregano Oil helps to remove calcification from the pineal gland, in addition to detoxification of the endocrine system. It is commonly used as an herb to flavor meats and pasta. It helps the immune system and acts as a natural antibiotic against infections and newly forming calcification. It is also used to treat foot and nail fungus, warding off insects, killing parasites, alleviating sinus infections and colds, sore throats, urinary tract infections, respiratory infections and yeast infections. It is also know to relieve bug bites, rashes and even poison ivy rashes, helps with cold sores, dandruff, and skin conditions. Also relieves muscle and joint pain, rheumatoid arthritis, sprains and cramps.

Coconut Oil revitalizes the brain and body and detoxes the pineal gland. It is thought to prevent Alzheimer's disease with medium-chain triglycerides that are converted to ketones in the liver, which restores neurons and improves nerve function in the brain.

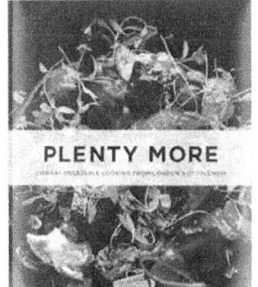

Tamarind fruit helps expel fluoride through the urine. It can be added to your favorite tea or used as a secret paste ingredient in your cooking. Yotam Ottolenghi is a great vegan chief who uses this paste in everything that you can find in his book called Plenty More: Vibrant Vegetable Cooking from London's Ottolenghi.

Tamarind is a common ingredient an Indian cooking and is used all over the world, including Middle Eastern, Mediterranean and Asian cooking. Tamarind is very potent, so a little goes a long way.

Neem Extract Oil helps to remove calcification from the Pineal Gland, in addition to purifying the endocrine system. This has been used in India for centuries. The entire plant is often used and ground to kill viruses, fungi and microorganisms. It is also known to help with arthritis, skin health, oral health, and diabetes.

Alfalfa Sprouts helps to detoxify the body, stimulate the pineal gland and provider a significant brain boost.

Chiorella is a chlorophyll and nutritionally dense superfood that removes heavy metal toxins, repairs damaged cells, declassifies the Pineal Gland, increases oxygen levels, boosts brain function, improves liver function, improves immune function, helps with energy levels, helps you feel younger, helps with skin tone and looks, helps with eyesight, helps with digestion, helps with aches and pains, and helps maintain healthy blood sugar levels. It is one of the few plant sources for vitamin B12, making it ideal for vegetarians.

Cilantro, also known as "Chinese Parsley" helps with mercury and heavy metal detoxification and removes the toxins from the brain and body into the urine. It also helps with diabetes, sleep quality, pathogens, anxiety and lowers blood sugar levels and oxidative stress and can prevent cardiovascular damage.

Garlic is rich in enzymes that dissolve calcium deposits. It also acts as an antibiotic that supports your immune system. It helps combat sickness, including the common cold. It can reduce blood pressure, improve bone health, improve cholesterol levels, helps you live longer, and helps prevent Alzheimer's disease. For best results, consume several cloves daily or crush the garlic and soak in raw apple cider vinegar or lemon juice as dressing for a salad.

Goji Berries is a happy fruit with powerful anti-aging and longevity properties, including restoring sexual function, improved metabolism, improving sleep, improving eyesight, and restoring glandular function, improving immune function and help promote health skin.

Gotu Kola is an herb that helps to nourish the brain and stimulates the pineal gland. It has been used for centuries to treat psychiatric disorders and physical problems, including improved anxiety, depression, insomnia, fatigue, Alzheimer's disease, libido, intelligence, longevity and memory. It also helps the body heal wounds and trauma, enhances the immune response, and improves circulation including varicose veins. For best results, drink Gotu Kola tea, but supplements are also available.

Hemp Seeds is loaded with well-balanced essential nutrients rich in chlorophyll and lecithin that helps brain tissue and supports the liver, making it a superfood of choice. It promotes cardiovascular health and hormonal balance and improves conditions including ADHD, breast pain, diabetes, heart disease, high blood pressure, multiple sclerosis, obesity, premenstrual syndrome, rheumatoid arthritis and skin allergies.

MSM – Methylsulfonylmethane is organic Sulphur, essential for a youthful and energetic lifestyle, helps decalcify the pineal gland, detoxifies the body, is necessary for collagen production for skin flexibility and complexion, is highly effective for joint flexibility, strengthens hair and nails, accelerates healings, increases energy, and works as an inti-inflammatory. For best results, work your way to a high dosage of 10,000mg to 20,000mg for several days accompanied with 1000mg of vitamin C, then drop the dosage to recommended levels.

Nigella Sativa is a black seed herb from Asia that is high in crystalline nigellone and amino acids that is shown to be an effective detoxifier, cleanser, antibiotic, anti-bronchial, anti-inflammatory that supports the pineal gland and immune response. It helps with type 2 diabetes, epilepsy, colon cancer, breast cancer, brain cancer, oral cancer, leukemia, brain damage from lead, some bacterial infections, and protects against heart attach damage.

Parsley helps to detoxify heavy metals, cleanses the body, stimulates the pineal gland, neutralizes the EBV virus, improves the immune system and helps with energy levels.

Zeolite is a natural detoxifier that will remove calcium shells around the pineal gland; it is also an effective environmental and heavy metal detoxifier, slows the growth of cancer cells, is effective against pathogens, and supports the immune system.

Dry Sauna's for a period of time can help to excrete sodium fluoride from fatty tissues, along with other toxic substances, with significant improvement to thyroid function, blood pressure, oxygen uptake, balance, reaction time and even IQ rating. Aside from making you feel good, it can help significantly with chronic fatigue, depression, arthritis, congestive heart failure, and pain and skin conditions.

Alkaline foods can help with detoxification of the pineal gland, reduces stress and improves your overall energy. Acidic foods draw alkaline nutrients and minerals from the body to neutralize the effect, which can lead to a buildup of acids in the cells and further calcification. Diseases favor an acidic state, so with the onslaught of acidity from stress and diet, balance is needed to maintain health and more focus on your alkaline intake is needed to fight disease.

Human blood pH should be somewhat alkaline between 7.35 and 7.45. Anything below or above this range suggests systems of disease. A pH balance of 7.00 is neutral, below that is acidic and above that is alkaline. Common causes of acidity include toxic overload, stress, and immune reactions that deprive the cells of oxygen and ability to absorb nutrients and minerals.

Diets consisting of 50% alkaline forming foods are recommended to maintain health. To restore health and promote decalcification of the pineal gland, diets of at least 75% alkaline are suggested.

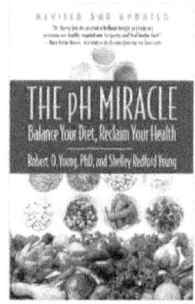

Dr. Robert Young book: The pH Miracle: Balance Your Diet, Reclaim Your Health, explains why you should never count calories, fat grams, or portion sizes ever again. The body's pH balance is the key to optimal weight, mental clarity, and overall vigor. Say good-by to low energy, poor digestion, extra-pounds, aches and pains, and disease.

Complete coverage of core nutrients, cleansing, exercising right, and alkaline foods.

Although many fruits are acidic, most are actually alkaline-forming in the body.

Amongst the best alkaline forming foods to eat are fresh fruits, green vegetables, nuts and seeds.

Highly alkaline forming foods include baking soda, lime, lemons, lentils, lotus root, mineral water, nectarine, onion, persimmon, pineapple, pumpkin seed, raspberry, sea salt, sea vegetables, seaweed, sweet potato, tangerine and watermelon. Fresh lemonade and watermelon are particularly effective for detoxification of the pineal gland.

Alkaline based homemade juices are highly effective.

Chlorophyll-rich Superfoods such as blue-green algae, chlorella, spirulina, and wheatgrass help to detoxify the pineal gland with strong cleansing properties. They offer similar benefits of leafy green vegetables in a much smaller serving.

Raw Apple Cider Vinegar is rich is malic acid and helps alkalize the body, it's a great way to detoxify and decalcify the body. You can have it straight up or with a glass of water, lemon juice, honey, tea or as a salad dressing. For best results, take before meals, anywhere from 1 to 3 teaspoons, 1 to 2 times daily, when choosing a brand, make sure it is in a bottle rather than plastic, raw, organic and has "The Mother" in it.

Extremely acidic foods include alcohol, artificial sweeteners, beef, beer, breads, brown sugar, carbonated soft drinks, cereals , chicken, chocolate, cigarettes, coffee, custard, deer, eggs, fish, flour, fruit juices with sugar, grains, jams, jellies, lamb, maple syrup (processed), meats, pasta (white), white flour, pickles (commercial), pork, seafood, sugar (white), table salt (refined and iodized), tea (black), turkey, white bread, white vinegar (processed), whole wheat foods, wine, and yogurt (sweetened).

Acidic fruits are blueberries, canned fruits, glazed fruits, cranberries, currants, plums, prunes.

Acidic vegetables are corn, lentils, olives and winter squash.

Acidic nuts include cashews, legumes, peanut butter, peanuts, pecans, tahini, and walnuts.

There are a wide range of resources on the internet to review alkaline foods and recipes.

Alkaline Food Lists
https://www.google.com/search?q=alkaline+foods+list

Alkaline Food Recipes
https://www.google.com/search?q=Alkaline+Food+Recipes

You can't roll black time with fluoride intake, but there are many ways you can restore pineal gland function and detoxify your body to restore youth, vitality, and health while increasing your range of conscious expressions and experiences.

The Childhood Awakening

Children before puberty have access to a wider range of conscious expressions than adults. They are often more intuitive, can tell what their parents are thinking about and to some extent can even foresee future events. At about age 8, the pineal gland function diminishes and the pituitary gland becomes dominate, resulting in reduced melatonin and increased serotonin production, changing the dynamics and ranges of conscious perception, imagination and childhood play, to more of a sexual awakening, starting to mature from the mystical childhood to the rational adult.

The New Age movement and some self-help teachings are based on getting you back to that childhood like wonder. Until puberty, fantasy and reality blur together. Children have a natural psychedelic and hallucinogenic state that allows them to fantasize and even have imaginary playmates.

Those who awaken may have similar experiences, such as being able to see fairies flying around. This is usually attributed to naturally forming DMT – dimethyltryptamine molecules that target the same receptors as serotonin.

Although this might be an interesting journey, fantasy is a nice place to visit, but you wouldn't necessary want to live there, and there is so much more to your awakening to experience. Naturally forming DMT is also essential for vivid and lucid dreaming, along with day dreaming.

As for psychedelic drugs including synthetic DMT, LSD, Psilocybe Mushrooms, Peyote or even drinking Ayahuasca goes, this may enhance your experience, but you are much more likely to have a bad trip with a drug than with your own naturally occurring DMT.

A few months ago, I was sitting on the couch with my 4 year old grandson watching a cartoon movie. I had one leg crossed over the other with my left foot hanging over my right leg. I decided to do an experiment... I manifested some Shakti orange Cheetos on my left leg. Within a few minutes, my grandson reached over and picked one up with his two fingers, started holding it up in the air, looking at it from various angles. He finally threw it to the ground and wiped his fingers on his shirt.

Now I've come a long way since my awakening several years ago, can do many things like manifest Shakti objects, cultivate great subtle bodies as if they were herb gardens, and have come up with an incredible energy ball for nailing juvenile delinquents right upside the head, but never once have I thought about picking up a Shakti object, never mind moving it around with my hand. I don't even have the faintest neural pathways to begin to do that, and here my grandson is showing me up without even thinking about it.

He had fluoride in his formula and then fluorinated town water, so I was somewhat concerned that it might impair his development. It hasn't yet, but calcification isn't really supposed to occur until later in your adult life anyway.

I had a talk with his mom when she was asking about the formula, but somehow I got outvoted. I had a similar talk with her when she was 16 and wanted to become a vegan. My concern was that it would stunt her growth, but once again she did what she wanted. Every now and then it becomes the joke of conversation that she is two inches shorter than her sister and could have been taller.

Anyway, awaking the pineal gland is like restoring your childhood ranges of consciousness and imagination. Once you have done it, there is no going back. It's like never having a large colored TV with all the channels, so you would never miss it, even if you heard about it or saw it in action at a friends or in a store, you would just be content going home to your small black and white screen, with bunny ear antennas, that need adjusted every time you try to change the channel.

However, once you remember what consciousness was like when you were a kid, or are fortune enough to revisit it for yourself as an adult, it's like having that color TV and you would never do without it again.

The Pineal Gland "Third-Eye" Activation

Over the years I've done regular detoxification protocols, homemade juicing and have mostly been drinking well water for my adult life, so I didn't spend as much time trying to decalcify my pineal gland before activating it. My awakening was somewhat gradual over several months. Vitamin D deficiency, pesticides and fluoride toothpaste were the biggest things I've been exposed to. A healthy lifestyle should be able to cope with that, but I've recently decided to go back to basics and spend more time on decalcification to help bring my awakenings along even further.

The approach was simple; I decided to shake things up with a shock-and-awe activation of the pineal gland, using mostly theta vibrations, meditations and music.

It worked all too well, including being able to sleep better, dream in color again, and have frequent vivid and lucid dreams. Lucid dreams are dreams that you are conscious for, can tweak the story line, and have an easy time remembering afterwards.

Since my activation, I've increasingly gotten better at being able to see Shakti flora and cosmic energy everywhere; including what shape most people's subtle bodies are in, along with seeing their aura, as more of a pseudo "5th Dimensional" or "Shadow Universe" experience, which I've come to recognize as duality between ordinary matter and Dark Matter.

This activation also improved my ability to manifest and tune into my subtle body and its cosmic energies. Some people experience increased creativity and imagination too, but I've always done fairly well in those departments.

Before long I realized that all it takes is a deep desire to make you a magnet for people, situations and events, often with helpful coincidences occurring, along with an abundant boost of energy needed for any situation.

It is a first step to greater access to the cosmic consciousness in the form of intuition, inspiration, creativity, and imagination. Since most problems have existing solutions somewhere, with better access to the cosmic consciousness, more possibilities will effortlessly come to you.

It also opens the door to greater spiritual awakenings, astral awakenings, psychic awakenings and even sexual awakenings; see the appropriate sections of this guide for further details. Some of these awakenings may occur immediately and spontaneously, while others will need to develop over time or as you put some effort into developing them.

It also makes astral projection possible, connecting you to alternate plains of existence where time and space doesn't exist, allowing you to transcend your physical body and have "out-of-body" experiences, anytime as pseudo "5th Dimensional" adventures. This didn't come naturally to me, so it's something I continue to work towards and the main reason I'm getting back to basics to achieve higher awakenings.

What you need to understand is there isn't one single awakening. Although the pineal gland is the key and most common chakra that needs jump started, there are numerous awakenings on different plains, each having many levels of awareness, so don't assume your initial awakening is as far as you are capable of progressing.

Here are a few of my favorites for a shock-and-awe approach:

The Secret Genius Accelerator
https://www.youtube.com/results?search_query=The+Secret+Genius+Accelerator

Light Body Attraction – Pineal Gland Activation Frequency
https://www.youtube.com/results?search_query=Light+Body+Attraction+Pineal+Gland

Journey into Frequency – Pineal Gland Meditation
https://www.youtube.com/results?search_query=Journey+into+Frequency+%E2%80%93+Pineal+Gland

3rd Eye Chakra Awakening Solfeggio and Binaural Beats
https://www.youtube.com/results?search_query=3rd+Eye+Chakra+Awakening

DNA Activation MerKaBa Ascension
https://www.youtube.com/results?search_query=DNA+Activation+MerKaBa+Ascension

Pineal Gland Activation
https://www.youtube.com/results?search_query=Pineal+Gland+Activation

See the Vibrational Energies section of this guide for more choices.

You can also try s chemical stimulation of the pineal gland to activate it.

Raw Cacao is a highly prized bean by Indians throughout South America. It stimulates the pineal gland and helps to detoxify it largely because of the high antioxidant content.

Noni Juice stimulates pineal gland cells, neurological function, serotonin and melatonin secretion, resolving depression and insomnia. It also normalizes blood sugar levels, shrinks prostate glands, reduces cramping, heals digestive problems, clears inflammatory conditions, clears repertory problems, clears skin conditions, and reverses cardiovascular issues, high blood pressure, Multiple Sclerosis and Parkinson's disease.

Chaga Mushrooms are powerful for pineal gland activation, mainly because it is a hearty plant with high melanin content that stimulates the pineal gland while allowing it function more effectively. It is a very high source of antioxidants, helps balance the immune response, and helps prevent cancer as well as many other diseases.

Another technique for pineal gland activation is Yoga Nidra and Third-Eye Mediation

Yoga Nidra and Third-Eye Mediation is a healing technique practiced by yogis for centuries, starting with alpha brainwaves and progressing to theta brainwaves, it helps to relieve stress, increases longevity, prevents illness, improves health, improves awareness, and helps you tap into your intuition, creativity and abundance while achieving the deepest relaxation.

As Gurudev puts it, "Unburden yourself so much that you can pass from moment, to moment, to moment".

Amrit Yoga Institute
http://www.amrityoga.org/more-teachings/thirdeye-meditation.html

Amirit Yoga Third-Eye Meditation
https://www.youtube.com/results?search_query=Yoga+Nidra+Third-Eye

Amirit Yoga Guided Meditation
https://www.youtube.com/results?search_query=yoga+nidra+guided+meditatio

The Kundalini Activation

Raising your kundalini is generally easier than activating your pineal gland. You can use the same techniques and meditation to do so, just focus on your kundalini rather than your third-eye chakra.

Achieving ascension of the kundalini through the chakra system leads to different levels of awakening and mystical experience, until ultimately reaching spiritual awakening.

You may find that it happens spontaneously on its own too. Once the demand for cosmic energy (Shakti vapor) increases in the brain, the body will accommodate, and raise your kundalini; which is actually a tornado like force originating from your root chakra that will stir your subtle body, making cosmic energy much more abundant and available to the brain, endocrine system, and chakra system.

Another technique you can try is deep breathing; take it in through your noise all the way down to your diaphragm, slowly exhaling through the mouth. Try this in conjunction with theta brainwave entrainment and meditations.

While doing these breathing exercises, imagine you are not just breathing through your nose, rather breathing with your entire body, circulating through your entire body, and exhaling through your mouth. You can also isolate certain parts of your body, like each of your chakra centers, especially the root chakra, and imagine the breathing taking place through there.

Another technique is Kundalini Yoga Meditation:

Kundalini Yoga Meditation strives to achieve a wide range of conscious states through the alteration of brain chemistry and rejuvenation of the endocrine system. This awakening of the kundalini enables the ancient vital energy throughout the chakras, where the "crown chakra" is awakened, achieving the highest stages of Samadhi.

Kundalini Yoga Meditation
https://www.youtube.com/results?search_query=Kundalini+Yoga+Meditation

Merlin's Cave Activation

Merlin's Cave is a mystical place indeed. It is said to be a place of great power and true magic, ideal for manifestations of all kinds. It exists between the crown chakra and the third-eye chakra. You can use theta mediations to increase the energy of the pineal gland and you can raise your Kundalini to increase the energy of your crown chakra.

Each of these energy centers has its own frequency and where the fields of these two chakras overlap, a third frequency if formed. This third frequency is similar to what happens with different frequencies in each ear, resulting in a third frequency in the brain.

Unfortunately, this is just the begging of the quest for Merlin's Cave. Often when I do this meditation, I get a blue or green hue when my eyes are closed; suggesting one or the other hemisphere of the brain is dominant.

Every now and then, I manage to get all white when I close my eyes, suggesting harmony and balance. This is where the quest for Merlin's Cave begins, hidden in plain sight, hidden in the light, waiting for you to find the magic within you.

Whether you find your Merlin's Cave here or in your deepest desires, the journey is truly an odyssey of the mind and the wonder of these adventures will truly be mind boggling.

You will never know what you are capable of until you try, so when you ask God to win the Lottery, at least do your part and buy the ticket, and make sure your desires are known on a frequency she might actually be tuned into.

Taking an Energy Bath

Once you awaken to the duality of Shakti or pseudo "5th Dimension", you will quickly notice that your subtle body needs a bath. For the exterior of your physical body, it's more like grooming.

I had some film strung between my legs like some kind of a swimmer with webbed toes. I also had vine like things hanging from my physical body.

Having no experience whatsoever, I did my best to trim down this overgrowth. All you need to do is focus on what you want and suck it in to get it. Often I was pulling with my entire head to get it. One piece of this red film got lodged in my skull and was driving me crazy trying to get it out.

The next day at work I had a meeting with my boss. I was fixated on the red film in my skull and somehow was projecting that. Without saying a word, he seemed be able to sense the trouble, vaporized most of it and sucked it right in. I just smiled and said thanks. Clearly I had a lot to learn. This is like nothing I could have ever imagined.

Soon afterwards, I noticed a cashier who was grooming her customers. She took care of a couple of kids who were in front of me in line and then got something off my feet that I hadn't even noticed. I was really impressed, not only at the distance she was doing this from, but the mass of the objects she was doing it with, somehow taking it in with one small breath. This was all so strange to me, like a different world.

Soon I realized there was more to do than I first thought. I had some kind of exotic plants coming out of my upper body. The roots were like fish hooks in my physical body, with a steam that went up to a reddish balloon sort of thing. It was just a matter of flicking the roots though my physical body and they floated away.

Unfortunately, this was just the beginning. The internals of my subtle body were a bigger mess, with all kinds of Shakti flora. My kundalini was huge, suggesting my body was having difficulty with the solidity and overgrowth.

It's been a lifetime of neglect and chance to make my subtle body what it was and I really needed to learn how to make it better.

I started with a number of meditations to improve the energy flow and practiced selectively turning things to vapor. In time I got fairly good at being selective about what I wanted to burn off and expel, but I had a lot of help in that arena.

There are multiple layers to your subtle body too, sometimes with gelatin, toxic and bubble wrap layers that are meant to shed away or otherwise expelled. Mine of course came loose in my upper body, but was stuck in my lower body, sometimes causing vertigo as it flopped around.

I tried pushing this layer out in front of people, who were walking the other way to see if I could find any takers, but surprisingly most people would just duck or sidestep to avoid it, giving me a better idea of how many people in the city were actually awake or at least partially awake.

I did have two takers, one was a hostess and the other was a waitress. Both of them almost fell on their ass while trying to grab it and walk away.

I've also noticed a couple detached subtle body layers floating around the office at work. One was hyper active where you could feel it pulsating. These are generally loaded with Shakti life and sometimes eggs. I personally prefer microflora or some forms of plant based flora, and usually burn or expel everything else.

99

Upkeep of your subtle body is one of the most proactive things you can learn do to maintain an energetic and healthy lifestyle; achieve higher vibrations and further awakenings, while allowing the most ranges of conscious expression and experience.

Cultivating Your Shakti and Subtle Body

One of the first observations that I made after my mind-body awakening was that I was new to the game and more people than I would have ever expected were already awake at least to some extent. Those with the greatest experience include:

- Those who have been active since childhood and have more of a natural ability with Shakti and cosmic energies.
- Those who were brought up with Eastern teachings are generally more experienced with Shakti and cosmic energies.
- Those who live or work in the city have more experience dealing with a wide range of Shakti flora, but for many, that's not necessarily at a conscious level.

There was a lot to learn, so it was a good thing that I was a quick study. This can easily become a sink or swim proposition, hence this guide is to help prepare you for the kinds of things you might need to know and could experience as your perception of the Shakti world expands.

This is not exactly a survival guide, nor does it need to be a survival of the fittest situation, but it can feel that way at times, especially when even the basics are new to you and you find yourself in some challenging situations.

I had the good fortune, and not so good fortune, to work in the city, with a bunch of people brought up with Eastern teachings, many of whom were young and have been awake since childhood. Talk about being at a huge disadvantage.

A good mentor is helpful in the early stages, but be careful what you tell people, especially things like you are new to all this or you are not on your game right now, because you may find yourself in the middle of pranks and horseplay.

During the day, many of these people would resonate their subtle bodies, raise their energy fields, expel Shakti flora, causing others to spontaneously do so too.

The atmosphere in the office was often so thick with Shakti flora that you couldn't help getting exposed to it all. By the end of the day, they were all sucking it back in.

Every few days there was something new and more predominate in your subtle body to try, taste, feel and see what you could do with it. Different Shakti flora can give to new abilities to explore, but these usually only last as long as the Shakti flora does.

In some companies that I've worked, we would take breaks by starting fights with squishy balls. Here we nailed people upside the head with energy balls.

Some people have energy balls that you would need to shake off, which could easily infuse you with some good energy. Others have these powder puff balls that don't even penetrate the physical body and can easily be pushed away. Some have a very compact form of Shakti flora, usually dark green that they can fling like an energy ball. All of these can easily be redirected away from you, at another opponent.

Once you have a good gelation subtle body, you can extend it out of your physical body in a tubular fashion. Most people do this to be annoying, like sticking it in other people's faces during meetings to try and get a reaction, or wrapping it around others.

The first time I extended my subtle body in this manner was with some new guy in the office. He fired a power puff energy ball at me before we even met. It was perhaps the worst Shakti flora I have ever seen and I really didn't even want him sitting that close. I used my subtle body to infuse his, making him very sick by the end of the day, but better him then the entire office. By the next day he seemed fine and his allergies had even subsided.

Meetings are always interesting, you can quickly gauge how many people react to all the metaphysical horseplay and it's always fun to try and get reactions.

All of this can be as simple as attracting the energy of your deepest desires, being passionate about holding on to it, and if needed, defending the energy of your dreams at all costs.

You can also just leave it all to chance and take some time to explore and taste what the Dark Universe has to offer, until you find that special inspiration that resonates within you. Exercise can be good for beginners to improve their subtle body.

Most of this can happen at a conscious, semiconscious or subconscious level, with full awareness, semi-awareness or with blinders on!

Manifestations

Manifestation of artifacts, appendages, swords, whips, or just about anything you can possibly imagine is achievable with Shakti and the power of the mind. It's not a matter of doing; it's simply a matter of knowing it is already there. You can also conceive of something in a similar way that you would with a daydream. The more you focus on this holographic projection, the more sold it becomes.

Some people like to express their artistic side and pass their creations around for everyone to take a look at. Others curiously empower their creations, and desperately try to get them back if they are lost or stolen, as if they put all their inspiration into it and can't simply make another. The more solid a Shakti object, the more likely it will eventually get noticed by someone who would take it, as if they couldn't make it themselves.

Shakti objects don't usually persist without periodic focus, so generally you just create what you need as you have a need. As for sparing with opponents, a sword is great for decapitations, whips are best used on the eyes where you can get physical reactions, and appendages are great to wrestle with someone who is trying to unload something on you that you don't want.

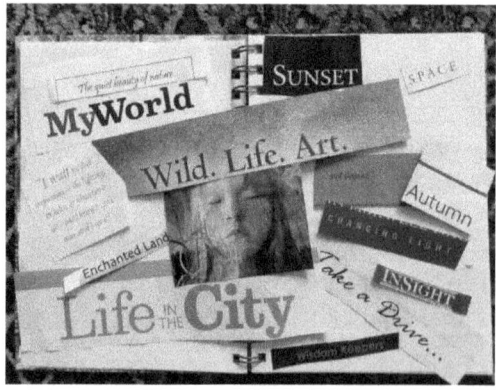

Lucid Dreaming

With lucid dreaming you are aware of everything around you, especially movement in a semi-awake state, so it is probably an evolutionary advantage to be able to do this.

You are actually in a very deep state of delta brainwave sleep that is difficult to wake from and can leave you dazed and confused if you do, so its often best to just go back to sleep. However, researches have found that lucid dreaming, hallucinatory dream activity, and wake-like reflective awareness is occurring at the higher-than-REM gamma and theta brainwave frequencies, which represents a hybrid state of consciousness.

The beauty of this form of dreaming is its easier to remember the dream, and take control of or alter the flow of the dream. This is perhaps the best way we have of exploring our subconscious mind too.

I do this kind of dreaming all the time, it just takes getting use to, but its more of a creative process than a learning process. I've had times I've written entire software systems in a dream state, but I can't say for sure that anything new was actually learned.

If I had to pick the most profound dream based realization for me anyway, it would be that in every conceivable way our reality is actually a duality. Polar opposites such as directions, emotions, particles-waves, matter-energy, etc. only begin to describe our reality from every perspective.

Nikola Tesla was a huge believer in the cosmic consciousness where knowledge could be downloaded "My brain is only a receiver, in the Universe there is a core from which we obtain knowledge, strength and inspiration. I have not penetrated into the secrets of this core, but I know that it exists".

Dmitri Mendeleev was looking for a logical way to organize the elements for months. One day he fell asleep at his desk while working on the problem, and when he awoke, the periodic table was born.

Alfred Russel Wallace traveled the world recording the species he found. He had an extreme dream in the shape of hallucinations caused by a tropical fever. The theory of evolution and natural selection had come to him in a dream by the time the fever had broke.

Rene Descartes built most of the framework for the modern scientific method. The basis for this method came to him in a dream.

Awake states of daydreaming, imagination, meditation and even trances are also achieved through theta brainwaves that can help access subconscious information that eludes the conscious mind, without the need to sleep on it!

Gamma brainwaves are achieved while awake too, it's just a matter of to what degree. Researchers associate high gamma brainwave activity with in-the-zone thinking, peak performance, exceptional intelligence, excellent memories and being happy and compassionate.

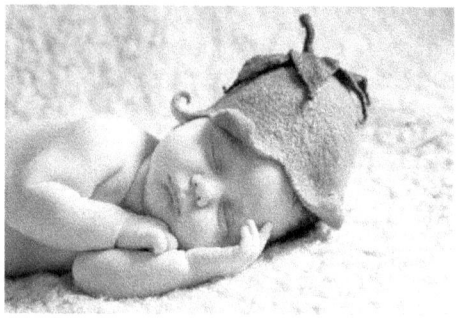

Out-of-Body Experiences

My sister as a young girl kept wetting her bed. She claimed she went to the bathroom so she couldn't understand it. Her grandmother finally told her to just remember to take her body with her, so she did and the bed wetting stopped.

Over the years I have been intrigued by stories of astral-projection experiences. I've often wondered if this was real or imaginary. To this day I still can't answer that, but in recent years I have been able to go out-of-body.

It's much simpler than you might think... With your subtle body, you can extend your tongue anywhere around or in your body, at practically any size. Going out of body is just the next natural progression of that, taking a layer of your subtle body away from your physical body, with your perceptions and consciousness being in two places at once.

I'm yet to venture very far, so I'm still wondering if this has anything to do with astral-projection. The phenomena seems to have less to do with spiritual or neurological factors, but more so Shatki physics that science hasn't recognized yet, similar to dark matter. Even so, I would like to think it is all related to spirituality more so than neurological.

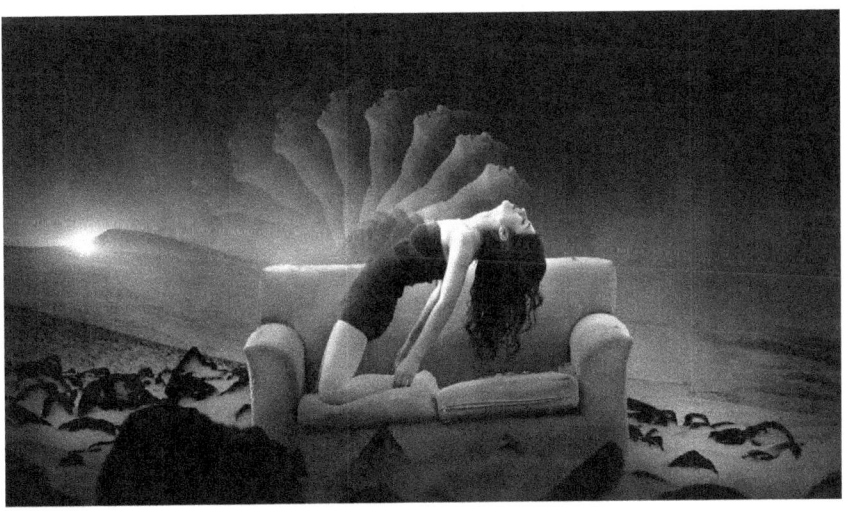

About Awakenings and Your Ego

Ego is often regarded as a sense of self-esteem, self-importance, self-worth, self-respect, self-image and self-confidence that serves to mediate the conscious and unconscious in a way that is responsible for reality testing.

This results in a personal identity of our own construction, with all the beliefs we have formed about ourselves, including abilities, skills, talents and personality, which dynamically grows, is self-reinforcing, and tends to lead to unnecessary emotional drama in our lives.

Developing a self-image is a normal part of growing up and maturing, but it can become inaccurate, overinflated, or pessimistic. Since much of this forms in childhood, it rarely translates to adulthood in a constructive and realistic way that truly reflects reality.

Many believe ego makes you feel superior, judgmental, arrogant or over-confident, yet in other ways it can make you feel inferior and over-critical.

There are several ways to know if your ego has too much control:

- You notice you are desperate to be right, not just on subject matters where you should be well above average.
- You feel superior gossiping about others and their flaws.
- You blame others when things don't go your way
- You get jealous when others do well.
- You talk about yourself frequently before even asking how others are doing.
- You frequently compare yourself to others, personality, looks, intelligence, money, etc.
- You have a deep need to win augments rather than just discuss different perspectives and ideas
- You have a passion to win anything at any cost rather than just doing your best
- You often sulk when you don't win rather than being proud you did give it your best.
- You beat yourself up for not being able to reach impossible goals.
- Nagging and repeating over critical thoughts

Spiritual awakenings often result in lack of desire, lack of suffering, and a clash with your ego that can take years to resolve. Once it does, the calm and collective mind prevails. Short of that, self-reflection is a good tool to use to help put things in perspective and help let you genuine-self prevail, or at least have more control.

If this is more than you are ready to commit too, now worries. The synchronicity awakening is a great place to be especially if you are young and single.

Chakra Cleansing

There are many chakras in the subtle body, but only seven are considered important. There are many interpretations of how the chakra's work, but they all basically entail the circulation of life-energy. There are some chakra's that are more significant than others for awakenings:

- Muladhara (root) chakra is essential for raising your kundalini (awakening).
- Sehasrara (crown) chakra is essential for spiritual awakenings and discovering Merlin's cave.

Chakra's are also essential for emotional energy flow and can become blocked, especially the Visuddi (throat) chakra. Here are some techniques and exercises you can do to clear your chakra system before proceeding further.

Try some breathing exercises; start with slow deep breaths in through the nose, exhale a little faster through the mouth. Now do the same thing while focusing on each of your chakras, as if breathing in from them, repeated several times.

If you find resistance in the neck in particular, that's where you need to focus further sessions, and you may need to breath in rather hard from the neck to become more aware of the blockage and eventually clear it. You can also try vaporizing any blockage with each breath. Also, you can try breathing past the blockage, just focus somewhere else in your body like the center of your chest and breath in from there.

There is a lot of information under kundalini awakenings and the appendix about pranayama along with Prana and Shakti.

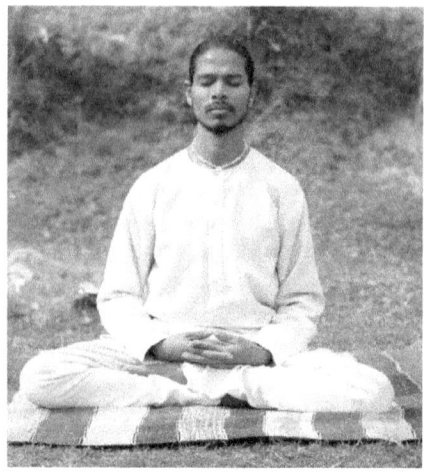

You can search the web to find a wide range of techniques for emotionally clearing this chakra, including everything from a massage to drinking water.

For more of an emotional chakra cleansing, try simply focusing on the color blue throughout your body during meditation.

Focusing on the color blue spiritually should help to increase calmness, peace, love, honesty, kindness, truth, inner peace and emotional depth. Green can work too, as balance, harmony, love and nature.

Kundalini Awakenings

In yogic tradition, kundalini is a primal energy based on Shakti, described as "coiled" at the base of the spine. The awakening involves moving this ancient vital energy up from the "root chakra" to the "crown chakra" at the top of the head, usually through meditation, breathing, or chanting of mantras.

Although this is essentially correct, let's take a moment to clarify what Shakti, Kundalini and Chakras really are:

In short, Shakti is the fuel that powers your spiritual growth and awakenings. The various cultural terms includes Hindu Shakti, Prana, Apana and Yyana, Chinese Chi (Qi), Polynesian Mana, Vietnamese Khi, Korean Gi, Japanese Ki, subtle energy and woo energy, Hebrew koach-ha-guf, Greek Bios, English Aether, Cosmic Energy, Kundalini Energy, Natural Energy, and Material Energy, American Indians Orenda, Ancient Germans Od, and Scientifically known as Dark

Mater, most of which are believed to be a part of any living thing, translating to breath, air, gas, or life force that permeates the universe.

In short, your subtle body has many components, perhaps the most significant is a lining around it. You can pull down more layers of this incredible material from your crown chakra. Each chakra, from the root to the crown, is a small "coil" on this lining that bunches the lining, and is used as a focal point to ignite and extinguish Shakti.

The kundalini itself is actually a pin at the top of your anal canal. This pin carries an electric charge, and is needed to maintain proper subtle body pressure and the tornado like effect that breaks down Skatkti into vapor for the brain.

To answer your question, you will become aware of your kundalini with an awakening, feeling it through your lower body, as a force that moves, and can be used to ignite other chakras directly.

Once your root chakra is ignited, your kundalini is free to start. You can use meditation to do this, just focus on your root chakra and kundalini. Perhaps the easiest way to ignite it is to do slow breathing to and from your root chakra, while focusing on your root chakra, which is just over the anal canal inside your body.

What can take years for some people to do the first time ultimately becomes so easy that you will be able to ignite any part of your lining with little to no thought at all.

This can be very exciting times, exploring all the sensations of different Shakti, however people who are new to this will have all kinds of Shakti in their subtle body. It also goes around like flora does in the physical world, so it's hard to avoid. In any case, some Shakti is like a bad drug, so its best NOT to burn some Shakti off as energy.

Variations on Pranayama might be helpful:

- Exhale quickly if you sense some form of Shakti powder or vapors that you don't like, especially if it tastes more chemical than living Shakti flora, or especially if it is too overpowering and feels like a bad drug. This will help to train your body to "smoke" the Shakti rather than "burn" it into vapors.
- Separate the prana in your mouth using your tongue, and then draw it up to your brain directly for relief of bad symptoms.
- With Shakti that is already in closer to a gaseous or vapor state, you can usually excrete it out of the subtle body all at once, or even give it as a gift by placing it in to someones aura.

109

Likewise, you can start and stop your kundalini as needed:

- To start it, ·breath in prana to each of your chakras below the throat, then just focus on the root charkra, breathing in and out slowly.
- To stop it, you will find you will be able to extend your lips to your root chakra or any part of your subtle body for that matter. Size really doesn't matter when you do this. Once you do, suck in real hard on the chakra to stop it. Suck only on the chakra itself and don't mess with the pin a short distance behind it. Keep in mind that it may restart spontaneously now, once your brain is use to this form of energy it will likely start calling for it as needed.
- There are people who can start/stop their kundalini along with others too with their mind. I'm yet to master this skill.

Each form of Shatki you burn will give you more of a perception of the world of Shatki, your subtle body, and may even reveal special and temporary abilities, but generally good Shatki will be clean and more like:

- Your eyes are clear and bright
- You have the power to take a full breath
- You feel vitality and full of energy
- You have a clear mind
- You have a good memory
- You have the ability to deeply relax
- You have the ability to fall asleep and get a good night's rest
- You face the stress with resilience and courage
- You have both an inner and outer glow
- You can easily digest life experiences
- You have the ability to expel toxins from your subtle body and mind
- You have fewer than usual emotions
- People are drawn to you more than usual

For the first four years of my journey, I strictly relied on my kundalini and didn't think chakras even really existed. With your subtle body, there is always more than one way to accomplish anything, but its best to keep it simple until you are ready for more advanced things. Eventually you will find you don't even need your kundalini or your chakras, your lining is sufficient to ignite Shakti anywhere in your body and can drop your body temperature by as much as a couple of degrees.

Another way to go is to focus on third-eye activation which may involve detoxification and decalcification. You may find that your kundalini ignites spontaneously on its own once your third-eye is active. Once the demand for cosmic energy (Shakti vapors) increases in the brain, the body will accommodate, and raise your kundalini; which is actually a tornado like force originating from your root chakra that will stir your subtle body, making cosmic energy much more abundant and available to the brain and endocrine system. This is actually the way I did it, with a spontaneous kundalini raising.

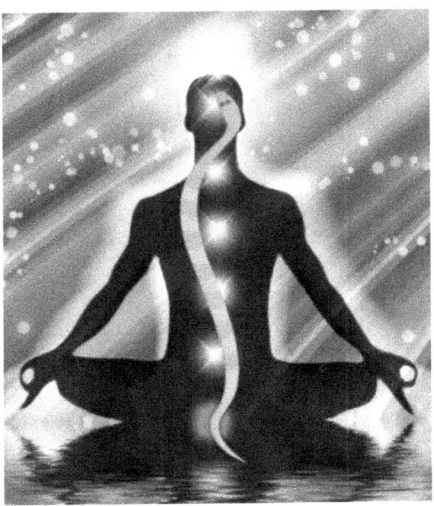

Third-Eye Awakenings

Third-eye activation may involve detoxification and decalcification. You may find that your kundalini ignites spontaneously on its own once your third-eye is active. Once the demand for cosmic energy (Shakti vapors) increases in the brain, the body will accommodate, and raise your kundalini; which is actually a tornado like force originating from your root chakra that will stir your subtle body, making cosmic energy much more abundant and available to the brain and endocrine system. This is actually the way I did it, with a spontaneous kundalini raising.

Your meditation should focus on the pineal gland itself rather than any perceived location on your forehead for a third-eye. That chakra is a little different than the rest and once you are ready for chakras it will be between your eyes. You can also try theta music to help jump start things.

Many people have naturally forming DMT: dimethyltryptamine molecules that target serotonin receptors are more prominent as a child. This allows kids to have natural psychedelic and hallucinogenic states and even fantasize about imaginary playmates.

The third-eye awakening restores this child like state by making the pineal gland more predominate over the pituitary gland, regulating the chemistry of altered states of consciousness, including increased DMT production.

Although the main purpose of the third-eye is to perceive what many would view as the astral plain (world of cosmic energy/Shakti duality) with daydream like perceptions, many go through periods of fantasy and imagination, from fairies to ghosts. This can be a pleasant experience or make you want to go back to the way things were.

Control and understanding will come in time. One of the challenges with the third-eye is to learn the difference between astral and imagination. This can be as challenging as understanding a dream at times, but it is mostly just more to nature.

This exposes previously hidden influences on your health, energy levels, and results in entirely new levels of socialization including practical jokes and even energy vampirism (usually just getting a taste), challenging your skills, constantly learning new abilities and how to better manipulate the astral plane. Depending on the people you work with or hangout with, or places you hangout, and especially use of public transportation, this can be challenging at the best of times, but eventually it gets very easy, and can be a real confidence builder.

Ultimately, this will lead to further awakenings, such as rising of your kundalini, synchronicity awakening, what many call a spiritual awakening, and even the potential to strive for enlightenment.

Often Hollywood and many others associate the third-eye as a culmination of many awakenings and a six sense. You will experience many awakenings, but things like synchronicity is associated with heightened intuition and awareness often thought to be a third-eye manifestation.

As for a six sense, it's apparent we all have many six senses that can become heightened with the experiences of various awakenings, but like the third-eye, there will probably be a period of getting use to these altered states and senses.

Having said that, I would do it again, but it's not for everybody.

Since the kundalini often spontaneously awakens, and many people start with the kundalini awakening first anyway, take a look at Kundalini Awakenings too.

For further details, see the seconds titled Pineal Gland "Third-Eye" Decalcification and Activation.

Synchronicity Awakenings

During puberty, the pituitary gland becomes more dominate, awakening your sexuality.

Sexual energies include an aroused mindset, physical energies like hormones and pheromones, stimulation of flora of all finds, emotions such as erotic desire, passion, lust and love, with the appropriate release of cosmic energy to support these higher vibrations, all set in motion together.

Most people are locked into a "3rd Dimension" mundane consciousness and only get a glimpse of the higher conscious bliss through sexual orgasms, so they already have an idea of its nature and intensity. Some have experienced the higher sexual energy that can rise into the body with a full body orgasm. Some have discovered the higher sensual energy that is an effective way to enhance intimacy through tantric sex.

Like emotions, sexual desire is an innate part of our physiology even once you awaken. Your sexuality has a metaphysical aspect with even higher awareness, magnified sensory sensitivity, and heightened attraction.

Attraction and arousal are really about what turns you on. This can be anything from looks, appearance, humor, personality, fragrance, and vibes. In a pseudo "5th Dimensional" or duality metaphysical sense, it's really more so about vibes, energy, and synchronicity.

This state is often achieved when you raise your kundalini and activate your sacral chakra, your passion and pleasure center.

Chance encounters and opportunities to meet the opposite sex become common place. Having others form an intimate connection, while playing a game of synchronous leg movement, occurs with ever increasing frequency.

You find unbelievably gorgeous women wanting to play a game of throbbing genitalia, with some able to give you an erection without pheromones, almost always resulting in prolonged gazing in each other's eyes with an open invitation to flirt.

Some women have symbiont life that they can place over your genitalia. It appears to be some form of plant life, with thick peddles covered in very fine bristles, giving the most incredible massage ever.

My first experience with this was with a women sitting next to me at work. After a while, I had a subtle body orgasm that was like a whole body orgasm with an explosion sending shockwaves in every direction. People at the other end of the office were saying things like "'what the hell was that". So much for a private moment, I didn't even know there was such a thing as an subtle body orgasm.

I've had a couple similar experiences with other women in the office, but that turned out to be a more private tantric afternoon.

Many people have a symbiont lifeform in the brain. Some resemble a cord with a rabbit foot like thing that roams around the room, but others have a cord with the most incredible and energetic lifeform I have ever seen. Although some people seem to have some control over it, along with having private moments with others, or tasting subtle bodies, I don't have conscious control over mine, so I can only speculate.

At one point I had some Shakti flora that smelled like violets. As I approached the elevator in a parking garage, there was a woman in town for what looked like an interview. I thought she might like this violet flora, so I expelled all of it into her aura. She immediately turned around, took notice, and started flirting.

Another time I had a red, soft Shakti flora that was going around the office. I was in the coffee area talking to a couple of people, when one guy comes in saying here is what you do with this one, fashioning a horse size penis. We dared him to walk around like that to see how many people notice.

At lunch, a voluptuous red head came into the deli, looking over the menu on the wall. I was standing behind her waiting on my order. It was all a matter of vibes, so I extended this Shakti flora from my genitalia to her crotch.

She immediately started dancing in place, turning me on in so many ways. This was the closest thing to metaphysical sex that I've encountered since my awakening, in a public place, in a very exhibitionist way.

There have been plenty of opportunities to flirt too, but with two very attractive women with strong vibes, I took my focus and very slowly moved it towards their crotch to see if they would notice. Both of them pulled their lower bodies back and started laughing, so it was all good, and it just goes to show we have a lot more than six senses. It has to be at least a dozen senses that I'm aware of so far.

Before my awakening, I thought all that was really new in the way of sex and 21st century was internet dating, smartphones, more open communication with texting, and arranged hookups.

Now, to meet that special someone, I wouldn't trade synchronicity for the all of the best and most advanced technologies on the market, although I'm sure synchronicity would work though these technologies too.

If you like the book, please take a moment to do a review of Destination Enlightenment at: http://www.amazon.com/author/danharp

Spiritual Awakenings

It actually started with health problems in my 20's from exposure to an environmental contaminate. As it turned out, I had to become very resourceful to overcome this problem.

The final part of the condition was a peripheral nephropathy that I was trying to overcome with mind-body techniques. After much struggling with this approach, it practically resolved itself once I learned how to raise my vibrations.

Other than health, I really wasn't trying to take things any further.

Then I simply awoke in a lucid dream, where I had these ancient ceramic plates with glyphs around the edges coming at my face, causing spasms in the center of my brain. I finally awoke from this out of concern it was going to cause brain damage or something.

All day long, I was looking around expecting to notice something different about reality, but nothing changed. In the weeks that followed, I was noticing an insatiable appetite for things I hadn't had any real interest in before, including ancient cultures, esoteric knowledge, meditation, and brainwave entertainment.

Within a year, I managed to rush through several awakenings, including third-eye, kundalini, synchronicity, which was a lot to get the hang of in such a short time. About a year after that, I had my spiritual awakening.

My spiritual awakening was rather spontaneous compared to the others, which were a little more gradual.

It started at work, where I found myself in a meeting with three other very highly charged individuals. I was mostly there to show a level of participation, so I wasn't particularly interested in the subject matter, and found myself getting mesmerized with the natural high of the moment, somewhere in the gamma range of frequencies.

A rift in space time appeared above me. It was an amazing energy wave accompanied with immense joy and bliss that I could only describe as heavenly sent.

I'm somewhat of a skeptical traveler when it comes to reading about spiritual matters that others have experienced, but here I was in complete wonderment.

This was the wrong brainwave frequency for third-eye and daydream perceptions, which are all holographic anyway. I've never once had a hallucination either, and couldn't explain how that could be accompanied with such overwhelming emotions.

That night I went for a long walk on some trails in the woods to reflect. After about a mile or so, I wondered into the woods though the trees until I was good and lost. I found a nice spot to take a break and found myself drifting off into a trance.

Instead of seeing a heavenly rift again, or being handed the keys to the pearly gates, I found myself going deeper into the trance, standing in an ancient temple, with some pagan statue surrounded by fires.

It was like stumbling on to a primitive part of the subconscious that I hadn't seen before, but instead of gaining greater access, or better yet a "root command prompt" to my own operating system, it came across as something that resembled a test with a bunch of questions, that I later realized was actually a very dramatic way of discovering my true calling, because at the time all I could really think of was WTF.

I began aimlessly wondering the woods until I finally came to a clearing. I looked up and saw Orion's Belt. I must have gazed at it for an hour or so. Dawn was approaching and all I could think of was home. Somehow I managed to come walking out of the woods into my very own backyard and have no idea how I found my way. I like astronomy, so I might have done some subconscious celestial navigation.

Other than the "how", I don't view any of the aspects of my spiritual awakening to be out of the ordinary from what others have experienced, although I'm still working on stabilizing everything and getting a persistent enlightenment going, which is proving to be incredibility challenging.

Sometimes the best way to find the path is to allow yourself to get good and lost!

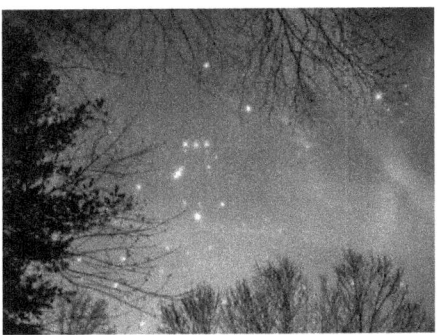

The "how" it all works is thought to result from gradually building a bridge from the physical self to the soul as we evolve and gain experience, often over many lifetimes. This energetic cord between the lower self and higher self is called the "antakarana", which involves the stimulation and building of threads to the heart chakra, throat chakra and crown chakra, allowing you to realize the soul's profound guidance, love and wisdom.

These connections, or conduits, are not natural and must be built over time with spiritual growth often starting from childhood. Developing this spiritual path is not done by doing, rather by being with higher purpose. This is an inner journey leading to the soul, while the outward life expressions are merely a reflection, or manifestation, of this inner journey.

Through meditation, one must detach from the physical, mental and emotional aspects of one's lower self to discover the path to the soul, transcending personality to discover the abstract mind, where the soul is found.

117

You can strengthen this connection to the soul by thinking and living in the abstract world, with things like love.

Although this connection takes a lifetime, your spiritual awakening is often just a matter of raising your kundalini to your crown chakra, at an appropriate time and with the right Shatki to give you the energy necessary for the experience.

My spirituality has developed over a lifetime, although my awakening was very spontaneous.

As John O'Donohue and Adam Cara put it in A Book of Celtic Wisdom, "Once the soul awakens, the search begins and you can never go back. From then on, you are inflamed with a special longing that will never again let you linger in the lowlands of complacency and partial fulfillment. The eternal makes you urgent. You are loath to let compromise or the threat of danger hold you back from striving toward the summit of fulfillment."

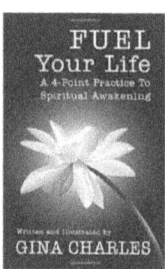

FUEL Your Life by Gina Charles points the way beyond the conceptual understanding of spirituality to find our power and learn how to live it, with authentic living perspectives that can be applied to anyone in everyday life. Live outside the limitations of unnoticed thought and role behavior. The life of your dreams is an authentic life experience.

http://ginacharles.com./

Astral Awakenings

In the broader term of an astral awakening, of relating to a nonphysical realm of existence to which many psychic and paranormal phenomena are ascribed and which the body is said to have a counterpart, the astral body, which can experience astral travel, known as astral projection, according to many cultures and belief systems around worldwide.

Astral travel is a separation of the astral body from the physical body, where the consciousness goes with the astral body. As it is called, a silver cord remains connected between your astral body and your physical body. Generally, astral travel occurs when you are awake without dreaming.

It not clear if out of body experience the same or just similar as astral projection. Out of body often isn't a conscious intent to do it and it doesn't usually last as long, sometimes being shocked by what has happened, but when done deliberately with distance from the physical body may happen more naturally by experienced travelers.

The only advise I've seen to do astral travel is to simply raise your vibrations to a very high frequency to get out of body and let go of any fear about leaving your physical body behind. It sounds like you need to achieve a frequency in the theta ranges that allows you to experience something similar to lucid dreaming while awake. Inexperienced people can just start with their tongue and go from there.

I have an sister that did out of body often when she needed to go to the bathroom as a kid. It wasn't until her grandmother told her to remember to take her body with her that the bathroom crisis was averted.

Recently I've managed to go out of body. This can be done while conscious, or in your sleep. I've only gone around the house so far, but what I figured out is you need to get your cosmic energy (Shakti) flowing well before doing this. What can happen over a lifetime is that this energy solidifies in the body, making it more difficult to out of body.

Psychic Awakenings

Psychic phenomena is often described as a non-physical natural force generally associated with telepathy and other metaphysical abilities, from the Greek term psukhikos "of the soul of life, spirit, or mind", meaning portrayed as psychic gifts.

Although everyone has intuition, not everyone has awakened their physic glfts, often referred to as one of our many "6th senses". It's not just a matter of having and trusting these abilities, you also need to express other transformations, like having a calmer quieter mind, while becoming a good listener.

Many aspects of this guide will help you develop your physic gifts, including a mind-body awakening, meditation, brainwave entrainment, and higher vibrations.

Telepathic and Empathic Abilities

Everyone has moments of telepathic abilities with everyday conversations, projecting thoughts, images and ideas in a discussion, which can be effective when all parties are on the same wave length, but this primitive form of communication is often dwarfed by its body language and verbal counterparts.

Thought is energy that can be directed towards others. Under the right circumstances, they will be able to perceive it, but depending on how it is expressed and their level of experience, they may not be able to distinguish it from their own thoughts; hence the "idea" that everyone has at the same time or the ability of using the power of suggestion in a subliminal manner.

Empathic abilities include understanding the states of others in social interactions, beyond body language, verbal communication, feelings and even thoughts that are directed towards them, otherwise known as mind reading. Scientists have been trying to measure the accuracy of empathic abilities for decades, but there is no doubt that everyone gets at least some moments of perception and vibes about others.

When I was younger, I found a wormhole in my subconscious mind, but was unable to explore it except in my dreams. I've seen a glimpse of the other side, but keep getting forced back, as if I'm not ready. It's hard to say how real this experience is in a dream, so I tried for years to explore it while awake.

About 20 years ago, I was at a conference in a large auditorium. At first I thought they were using some form of white noise, because everyone was mesmerized by the speaker. I started day dreaming, projecting holograph images floating in the air that I was able to view with my physical eyes. I haven't done that since I was in grade school, but even then I often found it easier to do around certain other people, probably those predominate in the theta range of frequencies.

It wasn't long before the guy to my left formed a stronger connection with me. Since he wanted to share, I decided to show him what I was working on, a wormhole. We both went on an exhilarating ride, real out-of-body experience, while being awake.

Unfortunately, he totally freaked out, went out in the hallway, complaining about me to someone else. This other guy walked back in with him and told him to just look at me. I was still mesmerized enjoying the speaker. He then sat this guy down several seats away from me in an angry manner. He proceeded to put one hand to his head, close his eyes, and was acting as if he was the one broadcasting the white noise.

For some reason, this annoyed me, so I shut him down, forcing his field back onto itself and project my own field to completely block him. It didn't take long before the cowed became more awake, interactive, asking a lot of questions of the speaker.

Since then, there have been many people who have tried to make a stronger connection with me, but those who I found annoying, I would simply take them for a ride in the wormhole. I've always gotten the same result; they freaked out. An out-of-body experience at incredible speeds just isn't for everybody.

About 10 years ago, I was invited to a learning hospital to meet two doctors and several students, to go over my case. They must do these interviews all the time, but for some reason the doctors were encouraging two of the students to be the center of focus and that we form a strong connection between each other. I played along...

As we got into more of an open discussion phase of the interview, one of the students wanted to know what I've seen, so I told her about the wormhole and we took a wild ride on it. She bailed too, but instead of freaking out, she found it exhilarating.

In the end, I told her that all that I have figured out so far is that life is about traveling; it's the journey that matters and the destination is merely a pathway to another.

All of this and much more have convinced me that even though the human ears cannot hear the range of frequencies used by the brain, we as a species have a way to broadcast and synchronize brainwave patterns. Even technology is now capable of generating waves or tones on the same frequencies as the human brain that can cause the brain to synchronize.

Several years ago, just after my initial awakening, I went down to the city with family and friends to see the sights. Later in the day, we were all on the subway. I was sitting in a separate car with my 3 year old niece who was sleeping in my arms. At one of the stops, 8 college students got on the car and sat in seats that were facing me. The odd thing was 7 of them were guys, all about the same height and build, but the weird part was their body language suggested they were using telepathy.

Before long, I had a "thought" that I could tell was external to me (from lower back left side of the brain), but it was expressed in a way that was supposed to make me think it came from me.

It went something like "wouldn't it be great to find a nice homosexual relationship right now", I replied on the same channel, "you know, that would be so great right now to find a nice relationship with a WOMAN!", except when I replied with "WOMAN", I cross circuited the right hemisphere of my brain and gave him both barrows at once.

The guy directly in front of me reveled himself by practically jumping out of his seat, and squirmed for a while before settling down again. Then I broadcasted "Dude, you have no idea what I'm capable of!". All 7 of these kids sat at attention in their seats for the rest of the ride, and the 1 woman who was with them just had a huge smile on her face and thought it was all so hilarious.

It's hard to say to what level telepathy can be taken, but the key to all metaphysical skills is practice, and with this ability, there is no better way than to find a small group of like-minded individuals to mentally exercise with.

Several years ago I was working on a project with many cross functional teams. There was a manager that they called the "hammer" who hounded and bullied many of the employees and contractors.

I was in a meeting with him, where he put his foot down with the entire group. He had a particular skill where he could make a statement while projecting an extreme emotional field, to the point where people would lean away.

I really didn't think much of his behavior, so I collapsed his energy field and used it to overwhelm the source, so he couldn't do it again. The rest of the meeting proceeded in more of an upbeat way without his participation.

Emotional energy can be projected (broadcasted) and channeled in a similar way as thought, although these frequencies have a Shakti and cosmic energy element to them.

Tele-Viewing the Past, Present and Future

Psychic awakenings are also associated with a "4th Dimensional" perception of time, to foresee future events or even perceive what happened in the past, in the form of tele-viewing.

Many of us have experienced close calls in cars, especially when road conditions were not at their best. Often the mind adjusts to these situations, so everything appears to happen in slow motion. Often people experiencing a pseudo "5th Dimensional" consciousness, and those having a really good time, living in the moment, find the mind does not perceive that much time has passed, when in reality it has. Although time itself doesn't change, the minds perception of time does.

Most people have experienced intuitive guidance about something that is going to happen. Depending on this vision, it can be exciting or scary. This may be a gut feeling, that little voice, or a feeling of just knowing. This instinctive vibe is either trusted or overruled by rationalization.

Intuitive awaking's expand your access to the cosmic consciousness, with a greater trust and wisdom that everything in your life is going to somehow unfold in the way that it needs to, connected to ones essence of higher self.

Several years ago I was walking into work and couldn't help notice very dark thunder storm clouds above and just knew we were going to lose power. I told a couple of coworkers that if there is anything they want to do in advance, they should take care of it soon. They were very obstinate, not believing me at all. Finally when I could sense the lightning strike in the distance, I told them "see, it's already happened", and they were like "what, nothing has happened".

At this point I just wanted to show off a little, so I told them "seriously, you know how this works guys", then proceeded to count down from 5 on my fingers, but when I got to 0, instead of saying anything, I just made my hand into a gun to shoot the light above. We lost power in that split second, and one of my coworkers was freaking out in his chair as if something miracles had happened.

Aside from already knowing we were going to lose power, from being able to tune into the storm (nature), sensing the energy of lightening, having a sense of how far away it was, and somehow tuning into the timing of it all, I'm sure it was nothing more than anyone who lived closer to nature could do easily, with skills developed over millions of years of evolution, that we for the most part have lost touch with in modern society.

As John O'Donohue and Adam Cara put it in A Book of Celtic Wisdom, "Your soul knows the geography of your destiny. Your soul alone has the map of your future; therefore you can trust this indirect, oblique side of yourself. If you do, it will take you where you need to go, but more important it will teach you a kindness of rhythm in your journey."

Men in Black III portrayed the first 4th Dimensional metaphysical character, named Griffin. A heightened ability to see what actions in the present can lead to probable outcomes in the future would do wonders for my trips to the casino, but more so, just the ability to tele-view the past would be incredible, especially since reality and the universe are often more interesting and fascinating than fiction.

Men in Black Film Trilogy
https://en.wikipedia.org/wiki/Men_in_Black_(film_series)

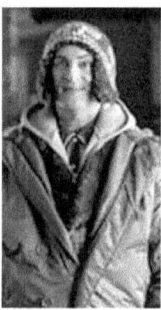

I'm sure if I had Griffin as a mentor on this journey, he would have something profound to say, like "We are in the midst of a great shift, an awakening of higher consciousness", "The day is approaching where we will be drawn into the light of understanding and spontaneous evolution", "Work with the past and the future while you remain firmly planted in the moment", "Time is always on your side, a force of nature that must be awaken within you, a force that is already a part of you, that flows though you and around you"

Achieving Enlightenment Persistence

Most believe they are physical beings, many believe they are physical beings learning how to become a spiritual being, probably fewer believe they are spiritual beings learning to live a physical existence, and at least some will believe all of the above. This probably depends on your faith, except for those who believe they are virtual beings.

It's not all about spirituality; there is an intellectual side to enlightenment, along with a very long rant about how there is a lot more to our physical reality, or should I say our duality, than you might be willing to believe.

In any case, a physical existence is the place to be for the young and is a great place to be for that matter. Exploring sexuality, starting a family, it's all good.

Becoming childlike again, with dominance of the pineal gland over the pituitary gland, including spiritual awakenings and enlightenment is a choice for some and spontaneous for others.

In any case, most spiritual awakenings can be very profound and can transition into enlightenment by giving your genuine-self oversight of your ego. Your ego needs to be tamed; you should also experience a lack of desire and suffering more naturally, and become more selfless in the process.

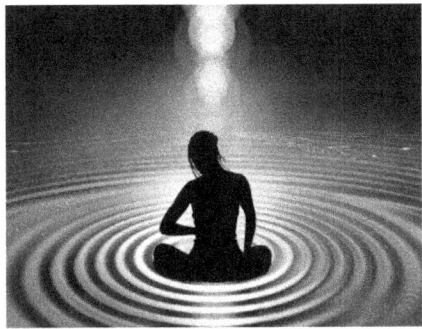

Enlightenment is only persistent for the very few who prepared for it.

Otherwise, you are likely to drop in and out of enlightenment.

Many cultures and religions do not prepare you for persistence. Quick paths like psychedelic drugs including LSD, psilocybe mushrooms, peyote and ayahuasca may get you a decent Spiritual Awakening, but any enlightenment will fail in time.

People who had spontaneous awakenings are also less prepared.

You really need to be in good physical health, have a handle on things like stress and anxiety, have a healthy subtle body, have a lot of experience working with the world of Shakti, are good at self-reflection to keep ego tame, can handle lack of desire and suffering, can make the time for all of this, and know how to defend yourself on various levels.

Once you backslide, you can get back to enlightenment again...

Under the hood, enlightenment is a distinct feeling or Shakti that your body produces. It doesn't make you all knowing, but opens your eyes in many ways, which can never be closed again, so in some ways it is persistent.

On the surface, it is a very clear and fast thought process with great visualization, rationalization and memory abilities. This can be lost if only for a while.

Most people probably think of it in terms of clarity, purpose and continued growth, so if you do have bumps in the road, you don't really need to start over again, but in many ways you will always be striving for enlightenment.

Once your kundulini is active, you don't need to raise it to your crown chakra; a much easier and enjoyable place to be for a while would be a Synchronicity Awakening to gain experience. For a spiritual awakening, make sure all chakras are ignited for a while until you experience something, such as a light from behind for several minutes to do a prayer. With enlightenment, you will need to work towards taming ego, desire, suffering, and selflessness. When you reach it, you will know the feeling.

In short, enlightenment is a lot of work to get persistence!

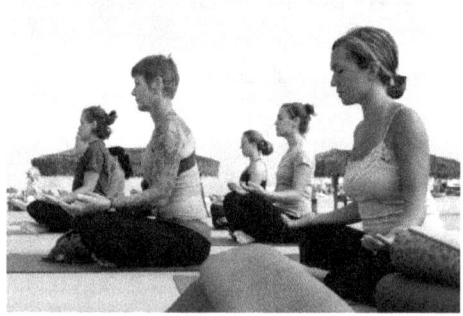

Chapter III - Power Tools for Your Tool Belt

Eastern, New Age and Personal Transformation Philosophies

Alexander the Great's vast empire opened the door to Eastern religion and mysticism to the west, while Greek philosophy and reason moved east starting around 340BC. This vast mixing of various religious and philosophical ideas has continued through the centuries, despite attempts from organized religion to suppress it, to reach a global scale and New Age.

The Age of Enlightenment followed the renaissance in the 17th and 18th centuries, was an umbrella philosophy meaning the emergence from self-imposed immaturity, offering education to the populace, freedom of speech and public debate, unalienable rights, application of scientific principles, the capacity for critical reasoning and freethought, often leading to much quibbling.

The Modern Spiritualist Movement has its roots in the 19th century, which became associated with women's rights, feminism, the abolition of slavery, mediums contacting the dead through séances and even scientific inquiry into the afterlife, with influence from the new thought movement, theosophy, and esoteric traditions and movements such as the Freemasonry and Rosicrucian's.

The Human Potential Movements started in the late 1960's drew heavily on self-help philosophies, theosophy, Zen and esoteric philosophies and took seriously that humans only use 10% of their brain.

The New Age free-flowing spiritual movement absorbed the Human Potential Movement and became popular in the 1970's, with a focus on spirituality, individuality, adopting beliefs and practices from a wide range of sources including Hinduism, Gnostic traditions, Neo-paganism, Wicca and Eastern religions including Asian mysticism, Shaman mysticism, Indian mysticism, Tibetan mysticism, Zen Buddhism, Secret Societies, Neopaganism, ufology, and the coming of the "Age of Aquarius", which is expected this century.

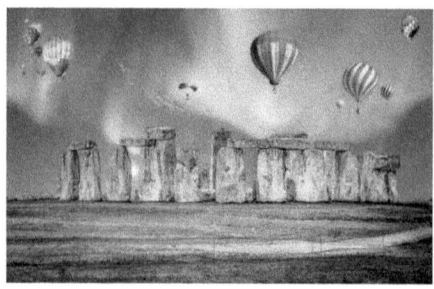

Although New Age is diverse, there are some fairly common beliefs and adopted practices. Practicing one or more of these techniques doesn't influence your religious beliefs, but may result in an alternate state of mind, personal growth, health, wellbeing, fulfilment, harmony with oneself and ones spirituality and could ultimately lead to awakenings that will change your perspective of the universe and perhaps even your beliefs.

- Individuals are encouraged to shop for the beliefs and practices they believe in and are comfortable with.
- Personal Transformation is a profoundly intense experience and awakening that leads to acceptance of New Age beliefs and practices, sometimes spontaneous or prompted by guided imagery, meditation, hypnosis, and even hallucinogenic drugs, with the hope of developing ones potentials, such as the ability to heal oneself and others, psychic powers, and a profound understanding of the universe, with some believing that when enough of us have awakened, a planet-wide transformation is expected.
- Meditating to release one's self from conscious thinking, often aided by a repetitive chanting or a mantra, or focusing on an object, sometimes with gentle, melodic, inspirational music.
- Aura is believed to be an energy field radiating from the body, detecting by some as a shimmering, multi-colored field surrounding the body that can be felt, thought to reflect state of mind, spirituality and physical health.
- Chi (qi/ch'i/khi/gi/ki) originated in China in the 1850's and has been adopted by many cultures around the world. It is believed to be a part of any living things, which translates to breath, air or gas, as life force, material energy, energy flow, vital energy, subtle energy, Prana life-giving force, or cosmic energy. Chi can form solids and lighter fractions form liquids, but most fractions are the life breath that animates all living things.
- Acupuncture is a part of traditional Chinese medicine that involves needles in the the body (skin, subcutaneous tissue, muscles) at specific acupuncture points to balance the flow of Chi. The practice often

involves burning mugwort on or near the skin near the acupuncture point.

- Zen is more of a way of like than a religion, an attitude or practice of heightening personal awareness through "zazen" meditation amongst other things, largely rooted in Buddhism, with Japanese and Chinese forms, which became trendy in the west in the 70's. It is regarded as a form of Humanism; human reason, morality, human and fulfillment.
- Reiki originated in Japan in the early 1920's and has been adopted by many cultures across the world. The practice uses palm healing or hands-on healing through universal energy that is transferred through the palms of the practitioner to the patient to encourage emotional and physical healing including spirts, mood, feeling, fame of min, temperament, disposition, nature, character, and intention.
- A belief in uniting to preserve the health of the earth; often looked upon as Gaia (Mother Earth) a living entity. People's allegiance to counties will eventually be replaced by a concern for the entire world and its people, regardless of gender, race or religion, and discrimination will finally cease.
- Reincarnation, similar to concept of transmigration of the soul in Hinduism, is a belief where we are reborn and live another life, which cycles and repeats itself many times.
- Karma, derived from Hinduism, a cumulate balance sheet of what goes around comes around, sometimes linked to reincarnation and how good of a new life you will have next time around.
- The idea there is a spiritual realm beyond the physical universe that interacts, however those involved in New Age rarely consider it a religion, never mind an organized religion.
- Since all is God, all religions are simply different paths to the ultimate reality. Some paths are harder than others, but all paths reach the same destination.
- All that exists is a single source of divine energy, or a belief in God being the entire universe and transcends it, or simply put that God is all that exists, seeking God within self and the entire universe, or that God is a higher consciousness that can be reached, or that God is a realization of personal human potential, etc.
- Various other practices and rituals are common, often to promote wholeness and balance, including astrology, crystal healing, homeopathy, chakra's, alternate medicine, iridology, massage, polarity therapy, ambient music, mantras, psychic healing, therapeutic touch, channeling, reflexology, foretelling the future with I Ching, Pendulum movements, Runes, Scribing, Tarot Cards, often to focus ones thoughts and mindset.

In short, the New Age movement is an amalgamation of freedom of religion and beliefs, gaining popularity largely due to the Internet, word of mouth, Eastern philosophies and other forms of media.

Achieving Zen in the Moment (Instant Zen Made Simple)

Although Zen will help make you feel more relaxed, that is basically a side-effect. The main goal is to stop wanting, which includes the desire to relax, a typical Zen paradox. The basic Zen principles includes no want, no desire, accept change as inevitable, live in the now, morality and meditation.

The Life philosophy of Zen is based on "The Four Noble Truths":

- Life is suffering, whether we like it or not, but are unwillingness to accept this is what causes suffering, in the way of not being happy with ourselves, wanting something we don't have, being irritated with others, or discontent with our lives.
- Suffering is caused by desire, because we want things, we wanting things to be different, we want something to happen or not happen, spending much of the say thinking about wishes, or we get carried away with these thought patterns.
- We must stop the desire, therefore, no desires translates to no suffering. Just simply let go of the pain in your heart about the things you need and live your life with what it brings you.
- Desire can be stopped by following the "Eightfold Path" where we learn to see things clearly and live our lives the right way. Desires will fade away and so will the suffering, simply by focusing on the here and now, Zen is best experienced rather than learned, with complete awareness though "zazen" meditation.

The "The Four Noble Truths" are achieved through the "The Eightfold Path":

- The Right View is the realization that everything in the world changes, including you, so clinging to the idea of permanent self is an illusion and gives rise to unhappiness; embrace change as unsettling as that might be.
- The Right Intention is to resist acting on feelings of desire, prejudgment, and aggression. Be sure of your motives, are they good for all or just yourself.

- The Right Speech is to speak when you have something positive to contribute. Don't tell deliberate lies, speak deceitfully, use harsh words to offend, hurt others, etc.
- The Right Action is keep from harming people, killing people, killing animals, stealing, sexual abuse, misuse others, or otherwise do wrong.
- The Right Livelihood is an honest life doing a job that helps mankind rather than one that is being harmful or just to get rich.
- The Right Effort means to reframe from helping or starting things that can cause harm or to actively help where good can be done. This is the driving force for others aspects of Zen.
- The Right Mindfulness is to focus on present events and do not judge or interpret. The ability to have a look at you from a distance, observe your body, feelings, mind without diversion. Keep an open mind in the present, quiet and alert.
- The Right Concentration is to reach complete concentration through "Zazen" meditation, which is an exercise to learn how to achieve the right mindset in everything you do and say to learn to see more clearly.

The basic principle of Zen is simple, that's right... life is simple and we tend to make it complicated. By sitting in the Zen style, or if you prefer try laying down, do some meditation as covered throughout this book, and experience Zen first hand. In time, it will all become more natural. There are many books out there, some keep it simple, many make Zen overcomplicated, so follow this basic Zen principle, embrace Zen and make it yours, but above all keep it simple.

The state of Zen can mean different things to different people, including relaxation or emotions like joy and happiness. In short, Zen is your place, that place you visit during meditation, or if you prefer the Zen tradition of "no-thought and no-images", it's really what makes you most comfortable, and it can be achieved in the moment with simple gestures, such as:

- Take a deep breath and instantly feel the calming effect run through your body.
- Take your hand, run it across your face and down your chest to achieve Zen in the moment as an instant transformation of your state of mind.
- Take a moment to envision everything around you is merely an illusion, and all that is in the universe is your presence, with an overwhelming feeling of being one with the universe.

Practice these exercises when you don't really need them, and you will be able to count on them when you do.

The "Just sitting" position is the very definition of Zen and is generally practiced with an "observation of breath count" exercise. This may take longer than a moment, but might be the best place to start for beginners.

There are three steps to this technique that is done in reverse order upon conclusion of the exercise.

- The Adjustment of the Body to achieve an optimal state of being free, which is a seated meditation posture, which should be the lotus-posture or half-lotus posture, but sitting upright in a chair can be substituted.
- The Adjustment of Breathing – start by breathing in through the nostrils and out through the mouth a few times. This is not complicated, strenuous breathing like yoga. Then start counting and bring each breath down to the lower abdomen. The idea is to influence one's mind-body to replenish fresh life-energy while expelling toxic energy.
- The Adjustment of Mind means to move to a conscious state of meditation and disengage one's self from the daily grind. It is generally possible to stop the mind by using the mind that is what the Adjustment of Body and Adjustment of Breathing are for, so in essence you simply detach and allow yourself to passively observe.

Japanese Zen emphasizes looking inside oneself to find the truth about the external world, understand the illusory nature of reality and become a better person. The logical minds sensory perception distracts us from seeing the true nature of reality. Dhyana concentration meditation is emphasized, giving insight into ones true nature, opening the way to liberated living, which is the state of no mind, achieving the state of perfect equanimity and awareness. Sit in the same place every day and the meditative mood should come by itself, like the flow of water in a river.

Another form of Japanese Zen is shibumi, which is overreaching in concept and ideal; simple, subtle, and obtrusive beauty; elegant simplicity, effortless perfection, effortless effectiveness, understated excellence, quiet refinement, great refinements, commonplace simplicity of spirit, appearances, noble and fulfilling in manner, and beautiful imperfections.

Shubumi is an understanding rather than knowledge, harmony in action, spiritual tranquility that is not passive, being with becoming, and must be found, not won. An eloquent silence and understanding that transcends knowledge.

There are seven basic principles to shibumi that can help you with any creative work, design or any projects, such as crafts, fashion, decorating, architecture, art, products, etc. that you set out to accomplish:

- Simplicity and elimination of clutter (kanso) – Eliminate what doesn't matter to make more room for what does. Beauty and utility need not be overstated, overly fanciful or decorative. The presentation should be fresh, clean, and neat.
- Austerity and irregularity (shibui/shibumi) – Reframe from adding what is not absolutely necessary in the first place; emphasizes restraint, exclusion and omission to present something that appears spare and imparts a sense of focus and clarity.
- Subtlety (yugen) – Limit information just enough for curiosity and leave something to the imagination. The power of suggestion is often more powerful than full disclosure.
- Naturalness (shizen) – Incorporate naturally occurring patterns and rhythms into you design; strike a balance between being of nature yet distinct from it, while seeming intentional rather than accidental or haphazard.
- Imperfection, Irregularity and Asymmetry (fukinsei) – Leave room for others to co-create with you; provide a platform for open innovation. Convey the symmetry of the natural world through clearly asymmetrical and incomplete renderings, which in effect allows the viewer to supply the missing symmetry and participate in the creative act.
- Stillness and Tranquility (seijaku) – Doing something isn't always better than doing nothing. It is in the states of active calm, tranquility, solitude, and quietude that we find the essence of creative energy.
- Break from Routine (datsuzoku) – An interruptive "break" is an important part of any breakthrough design. When a well-worn pattern is broken, creativity and resourcefulness emerge.

Meditation is an incredibly effective way to enhance self-awareness, focus, and attention for achieving creative insights.

Ultimate Tie Chi for Mind and Body Balance and Harmony

Tie Chi is a martial art for self-protection with much in common with Zen disciplines and the oldest form of Taoist philosophy, which is practiced with patience and skill, with a focus on training the mind as well as the body, achieving balance and harmony.

Movements are practiced very slowly and carefully to develop precision, breath control, balance, coordination, and internal power, making Tie Chi a gentle exercise with benefits including lower blood pressure, improved balance, improved coordination, better flexibility of the joints, improved posture, calmness of the mind, increased lung capacity, inner confidence, improved alertness, self-awareness, improved self-esteem, relaxation, and a clear and balanced perspective.

Wu Chi is the grand ultimate space where nothing exists, yet contains the potential for everything. Out of this rises Tie Chi, the journey from stillness to movement (extremes of yin and yang and back to stillness).

All Tie Chi form begins with stillness (Wu Chi), moves to the extremes of yin and yang in a flowing tide of continuous motion and comes back to stillness. An internal stillness is maintained throughout the movements of the form.

The interplay of yin and yang illustrates everything has an opposite, so however bad things get, the good times will come again, and when things are well, don't become complacent and appreciate what we have.

Meditation resting in the state of stillness can bring peace of mind, serenity and greater wisdom. This is a very powerful way to calm the mind and manage stress. This stillness can increase peripheral awareness, with is very useful for martial arts, along with mental stepping back and becoming the observer, making you better equipped to deal with difficult situations.

In many ways, Tai Chi is mediation in motion, which is aimed at reducing stress and improving health, helping you uncover the stillness with motion:

- Stand with your feet shoulder-width apart with your toes pointing straight ahead and your knees slightly bent.
- With your hips tucked slightly forward, keep your shoulders down and relaxed and your head held up.
- Slowly inhale and exhale deep breaths through your nose and your eyes closed or slightly parted and begin meditating.
- Focus on your feet and their connection to the earth.
- Use this meditation breathing technique: As you inhale, imagine that you are pulling energy into your feet from the ground or earth. As you exhale, you return the energy to the ground.
- Repeat this several times, then let the energy from the ground travel up your legs and into the center of your abdomen. When you exhale, imagine ridding your body of any toxic energy.

There are several variations of this standing meditation technique include seated, arms circled with shoulders down and relaxed, horse stance with feet wide apart (beyond shoulder-width), arms circled with shoulders down in horse stance, or opening and closing movements with your hands as you inhale and exhale.

When inhaling, think of taking life energy into your body. When you exhale, release that energy.

Tai chi is a means for deepening your awareness of and ability to relax on all levels of your being. The main emphasis of practicing an advanced method of Taoist meditation is to explore the nature of opposites, the nature of emptiness and non-duality, through rhythmic alternation between yin and yang with slow motion movement. The goal is a slow moving meditation to find and recognize the Tai Chi place in your mind where these differentiations come together and become one simultaneously within emptiness.

https://www.youtube.com/results?search_query=tai+chi

Harnessing Yoga Breathing Techniques, Meditations, and Practices

Although yoga is thought to be developed in India around 900 BC, seals were discovered in the Indus Valley Civilization of Pakistan that data back as far as 3300 BC that depict common yoga and meditation poses, that has evolved into many forms including Karma yoga, Dhyana yoga, Ashtanga yoga, Bhakti yoga, Vinyasa yoga, and much more.

Although yoga appears to focus on controlling the body, it is an ancient spiritual discipline, a form of meditation, harnessing breathing techniques and the energy of the body to tame the mind and passions, with assentation to various states of consciousness and forms of trance states that can be achieved by focusing on a single object or thought, such as a word or candle flame.

As an exercise, doing several poses, one posture (asana) to another, is said to help balance the body and soul.

https://www.youtube.com/results?search_query=yoga

The Eight-Fold or Eight-Limbed Path supports a life on integrity, spiritual growth, and physical, mental and emotional wellbeing, to learn ones purpose, to know oneself at the deepest level.

1) **Yamas – Ethical Code of Conduct**
   - Ahimsa – Non-violence in thought, word or deed
   - Satya – Truthfulness
   - Asteya – Non-stealing
   - Brahmacharya – Continence, moderation in all things
   - Aparigraha – Non-attachment, non-covetousness, non-hoarding
2) **Niyamas – Personal Disciplines**
   - Saucha – Purity, cleanliness
   - Santosa – Contentment
   - Tapas – Zeal, austerity, self-discipline
   - Svadhyaya – Self-study and study of sacred texts
   - Ishvara Pranidhana – The abandonment of the fruits of one's actions to a Higher Power. Surrender.
3) **Asanas – (Postures)** begin the physical journey inward. Asanas develop strength, flexibility, concentration and awareness and in the process make the body strong, healthy and fit for meditation.
4) **Pranayama – (Breath Control)** Pranayama techniques develop mastery of one's breath, a usually sub-conscious process is brought under conscious control. Pranayama reveals the intimate connections between mind, body, breath and emotions on an even more subtle level, allowing still deeper penetration inwards.
5) **Pratyahara – (Withdrawal of the Senses)** Pratyahara is the withdrawal from the outer world as experienced through our senses so we may journey farther inwards towards a more dispassionate, objective observance of ourselves.
6) **Dharna – (Concentration)** Dharna is the practice of making the mind "one-pointed", so as to steady it and make it still. This state of "one-pointed ness", when prolonged, leads to meditation.
7) **Dhyana – (Meditation)** is the state of existing fully in the here and now. Having naturally arrived at this stage thru the practice of "one-pointed ness", thought ceases and we abide in the present.
8) **Samadhi – (Bliss)** Union of the Individual Self with the Supreme. Samadhi is a profound state of grace that is gained after prolonged meditation, wherein the practitioner transcends the illusory sense of separateness from the Universe. Samadhi is the culmination of the practice of all the limbs of yoga.

Pranayama is the practice of a intricate breathing techniques in yoga and refers to several techniques for accumulating expanding, and working with prana in various disciplines.

Here are several effective Yoga breathing techniques. For best results, sit on the floor (Lotus pose) in the early morning or at sunset, or at least keep your back erect from the base of the spine to the neck, perpendicular to the floor on any kind of chair at any time, such as a break at work.

- **Agnisar Kriya Pranayama Technique:**
  - Inhale deeply from your nose while standing with your legs kept slightly apart. Thereafter you should exhale only from your mouth with your head kept slightly bent forward and the knees should be slightly bent too.
  - You should hold your breath for just a moment before you snap the abdomen backwards and forwards 10 to 12 times while holding your breath.
- **Anuloma Pranayama Technique** is about ultimate nostril breathing. In this case, the inhalation and exhalation is done with one nostril blocked and the other partially open; cleanses the nasal passages and bringing calmness within.
- **Bahya Pranayama Technique:**
  - Breathe in deeply (inhale) then exhale completely and hold your breath.
  - Try to pull your stomach upward as much as you can, pull up the muscles in the area below the navel.
  - After that move your head in down position so that your chin touches your chest.
  - Hold this position for 5 to 10 seconds.
  - Assume that all your negativity is being expelled from your body.
  - Repeat this process for 5 to 10 times.
- **Bhastrika Pranayama Technique:**
  - Take a deep breath (inhale) and gently breathe out, taking about 2.5 minutes to breath in and then out.
  - While you breathe in (inhale) imagine that you are taking in positive energy and vibrations, and that you are being energized by them.
  - During breathe out (exhale), imagine that you are taking out all the toxins from our body and find. (feel that during breathe out all the toxins comes out through your breathe)
  - Repeat this process for 10 to 15 times.
- **Bhramari Pranayama Technique:**
  - Close your eyes and breathe deeply.
  - Now close your ears lids or flaps with your thumbs.
  - Place your index finger just above your eyebrows and the rest of your fingers over your eyes with your middle fingers while applying very gentle pressure to the sides of your nose.

137

- o Now concentrate your mind on the area between your eyebrows.
- o Keep your mouth closed; breathe out slowly through your nose with making a humming sound of Om.
- o Repeat this 5 times.
- **Digra Pranayama Technique** requires laying down on your back rather than sitting, with deep in inhalation and exaltation.
  - o Breath normally and then slowly take deep breaths, relaxing your body.
  - o Now inhale a lot of air in slowly to fill your belly up. Hold this position for a few seconds and exhale drawing the belly inwards ensure there is no air left.
  - o In the second step, inhale deeply to fill up the belly. Inhale a bit more to fill up air in your rib cage. When you exhale, exhale air from your rib cage and then from your belly.
  - o In the third step, inhale deeply to fill up your belly and rib cage with air. Inhale a bit more to fill up your heart center with air. When you exhale, exhale air from the heart center, then the rib cage and then the belly.
  - o Repeat the whole process several times
- **Kapalabhati Pranayama Technique**
  - o Cross your legs and take two to three deep breaths to get yourself prepared.
  - o Now inhale deeply and exhale forcefully drawing all the air out. Your belly should be drawn in, as you exhale.
  - o When you inhale, let it happen passively without you making any effort as the belly goes back to normal position.
  - o Exhale forcefully again and continue doing this for about 20 to 30 times
- **Nadi Sodhana Technique**:
  - o Use your thumb (right hand) to close the right side of your nose. Inhale deeply using the left nostril. Now close the left nostril and exhale using the right one
  - o In the same way, now with the left nostril still closed, inhale using the right nostril and exhale with the left one
  - o Repeat 10 to 15 times per session
- **Shitali Pranayama Technique**:
  - o Cross your legs and take five to six deep breaths to get yourself prepared.
  - o Now open your mouth in a "o" shape and start to inhale through the mouth. When you exhale, do so with your nose.
  - o Repeat 5 to 10 times per session
- **Ujjayi Pranayama Technique** is about mimicking the oceanic sound or the sound of the waves for about 15 times per session.

- o   Cross your legs and take five to six deep breaths to get yourself prepared.
- o   While doing this, constrict your throat as if something is choking it when you exhale and inhale the air. This will produce a sound similar to the ocean when you breathe.
- o   Now close your mouth and start breathing using your nose, but maintain the same sound as your breath.
- **Viloma Pranayama Technique** involves pausing breathing at regular intervals and divided into paused inhalation and paused exhalation.
   - o   For paused inhalation, inhale for a few seconds and pause. Hold your breath for two seconds and then restart inhalation. Pause inhalation again after two seconds. Inhale again. Repeat this process untill the lungs feel full of air
   - o   For paused exhalation, do the exact opposite of the inhalation process. In this case, you inhale deeply and normally without interruption, but exhale with regular pauses.

Pranayama benefits include stress relief, reducing signs of oxidative stress, and improved digestion, autonomic function, concentration of the mind, tranquility, self-enlightenment, longevity and perception.

Dhyana meditation is the continuous flow of perception and thought, like the flow of water in a river. This should be done at the appointed time daily, when the meditative mood will come by itself without effort, with keen awareness without focus, to observe without judgement or attachment, while "contemplating" it in all of its colors and forms in a profound, abstract state of mediation.

Meditation becomes a state of being, with the line between what you are doing, such as breathing, mantra, light visualization, becomes blurred and the separation between you and whatever you are focusing on disappears.

The state that is reached where you forget that you're meditating - during Dhyana our thoughts, emotions and desires subside and our state of doing merges with our state of being... The subject and object become one.

Using Buddhism for Overcoming Suffering and Achieving Nirvana

The Buda strives to achieve serenity, compassion, generosity, wisdom, enlightenment, and spirituality to transcend the limitations of the body and break the cycle of karma and endless reincarnation. The path to attaining realization is often simply a matter of living as ordinary human beings reflecting on life's lessons, and to use meditation to enhance this reflection, often in trance like states, to obtain the supreme and ultimate awareness and wisdom of the universe; surrendering to nirvana, bliss, and awakenings that already exist within you, realizing the quality of every moment is what is most important while striving for balance, following the path to enlightenment on middle ground, without the need to learn the hard way with extremes, using this time, the energy you have here in this life, for your awakenings and enlightenment.

Who you are is constantly changing, like a river, with evaporation and rain to replenish, which is one way to think of ourselves in Buddhism. Compassion comes from understanding impermanence, transience, flow and that all things change; including how everything and everyone is connected, how one thing passes to other.

The Buddha's first sermon after his Enlightenment centered on the Four Noble Truths, which are the foundation of Buddhism. The truths are:

1. **The truth of suffering (dukkha**). The Buddha taught that before we can understand life and death we must understand the self. The nature of life is the nature of self. The meaning of "dikkha" is that which is difficult to bear, which can mean suffering, stress, pain, anguish, affliction, or unsatisfied.
2. **The truth of the cause of suffering (samudaya).** Become free of suffering by understanding the cause of suffering, living with the confused and entangling desires of our own mind, so be smart about your desires, without grasping, clinging or controlling every changing dynamic of your life. The Buddha's teachings on karma and rebirth are closely related to the Second Noble Truth.
3. **The truth of the end of suffering (nirhodha).** The Buddha's teachings on the Four Noble Truths are sometimes compared to a physician diagnosing an illness and prescribing a treatment. Beyond grasping and control and conditional existence is Nirvana. "The mind like fire unbound." The realisation of Nirvana is supreme Bodhi or Awakening. It is waking up to the true nature of reality. Nirvana literally means "unbound'.
4. **The truth of the path that frees us from suffering (magga).** Suffering and dissatisfaction is caused by our own mind. The noble eightfold path, consisting of moral discipline, mindfulness, and wisdom is a practice to lead the mind to enlightenment, intended to help make the path easier for others in a liberating sort of way. The benefit is not to merely believe in the doctrine; the emphasis is on living the doctrine, walking the path, moving

beyond the conditional responses that obscure our true nature, and moving beyond clinging to limitation, and attempts to control the ceaseless flow of phenomena that obscures our true nature.

The Noble Eightfold Path:

1. **Samma-Ditthi** — Complete or Perfect Vision, also translated as right view or understanding. Vision of the nature of reality and the path of transformation.
2. **Samma-Sankappa** — Perfected Emotion or Aspiration, also translated as right thought or attitude. Liberating emotional intelligence in your life and acting from love and compassion. An informed heart and feeling mind that are free to practice letting go.
3. **Samma-Vaca** — Perfected or whole Speech. Also called right speech. Clear, truthful, uplifting and non-harmful communication.
4. **Samma-Kammanta** — Integral Action. Also called right action. An ethical foundation for life based on the principle of non-exploitation of oneself and others. The five precepts.
5. **Samma-Ajiva** — Proper Livelihood. Also called right livelihood. This is a livelihood based on correct action the ethical principal of non-exploitation. The basis of an ideal society.
6. **Samma-Vayama** — Complete or Full Effort, Energy or Vitality. Also called right effort or diligence. Consciously directing our life energy to the transformative path of creative and healing action that fosters wholeness. Conscious evolution.
7. **Samma-Sati** — Complete or Thorough Awareness. Also called "right mindfulness". Developing awareness, "if you hold yourself dear watch yourself well". Levels of Awareness and mindfulness - of things, oneself, feelings, thought, people and reality.
8. **Samma-Samadhi** — Means to be fixed, absorbed in or established at one point, thus the first level of meaning is concentration when the mind is fixed on a single object. The second level of meaning goes further and represents the establishment, not just of the mind, but also of the whole being in various levels or modes of consciousness and awareness. This is Samadhi in the sense of enlightenment.

The Three Trainings:

The **first training**, and the indispensable basis for spiritual development, according to the Buddha, is ethics (shila).

Meditation (Samadhi) is the second training:

The Buddha taught meditation as a transformative practice to relax heart and wake to the moment, involving the body and mind as a single entity. Some methods involve concentrating on breathing, without altering the breathing, just be aware of the breathing, without thought. Other methods include concentrating n an object, candle flame, chanting mantra's, etc.

Meditation does not have to involve keeping still; walking meditations are popular using the Zen way of doing it, and repetitive movements using beads or prayer wheels are used in other faiths.

Meditation clarifies the mind in preparation for the **third training:** developing wisdom (prajna). The real aim of all Buddhist practice is to understand the true nature of our lives and experience.

Cosmic Consciousness

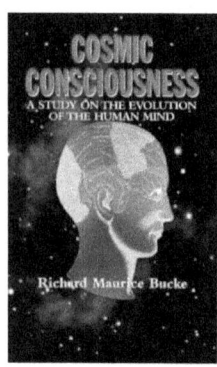

The Cosmic Consciousness was first described by Richard Maurice Bucke in his 1901 book, Cosmic Consciousness: A Study of the Evolution of the Human Mind. He defined cosmic consciousness as being "a higher form of consciousness than that possessed by the ordinary man". Becke proposed that his case studies with enlightened people were evolutionary jumps, the predecessor of a more advanced species.

Cosmic Consciousness Index
http://sacred-texts.com/eso/cc/index.htm

According to Bucke, "This consciousness shows the cosmos to consist not of dead matter governed by unconscious, rigid, and unintended law; it shows it on the contrary as entirely immaterial, entirely spiritual and entirely alive; it shows that death is an absurdity, that everyone and everything has eternal life; it shows that the universe is God and that God is the universe, and that no evil ever did or ever will enter into it; a great deal of this is, of course, from the point of view of self-consciousness, absurd; it is nevertheless undoubtedly true".

One thing is for certain, without some form of consciousness; nothing is experienced on any level. Science is yet to explain our consciousness, never mind a higher consciousness that is often perceived as intuition and inspiration.

Greater access to this Cosmic Consciousness would be like a high-speed Wi-Fi internet hot spot for the illuminated, but few have achieved that.

Does the universe represent God in manifestation and does all life collectively represent her living consciousness? Where is the exquisite quantum mathematics to answer that question?

Once science discovers and explains 100% of the universe in the form of Light Matter, Shakti and Dark Energy, they still haven't accounted for a living universe. This "Conscious Universe" is perhaps that portion of God's consciousness that is not in manifestation.

Although consciousness is needed to make all the probabilities and mathematics involved with quantum physics, the reality is there is no math to quantify or support its existence, only we can do that and see how far we can take it. As science explores the origins of consciousness, life, and its sacred geometry, we can experience it for ourselves and reach beyond the limitations of instrumentation to measure it, just to see how far the rabbit hole really goes.

As Hermes Trismegistus put it, "As above, so below, as within, so without, as the universe, so the soul…"

Esoteric Knowledge

Esoteric Knowledge throughout the ages has been put to use by those in power, who in turn suppressed it from the masses. This has always been much more than not allowing people to read and write. At least in private, it is accepted at the highest levels of powers today, that mysticism, which means "To Conceal", is alive and strong in the 21st century. In many ways mysticism, including alchemy is responsible for modern day science and chemistry, but the mystical experience has always been the realization of a higher understanding aimed at human transformation.

Even today we don't understand the full potential of the human mind, or even the best way to teach our children how to learn to learn, rather than just to learn by doing.

Mysticism and its esoteric knowledge may just be the closest thing we have to an instruction manual for "Awakening" the human condition, also known as "Enlightenment", "Bodhi" or "Illuminated" and experiencing the ultimate reality.

These ancient mysteries have been preserved through ancient cultures, religions, mythologies and secret societies. Much of the symbolism is hidden in plain sight, in architectures, rituals, traditions, practices, manuscripts, texts, and music, which is now available to some degree on the internet, YouTube and other forms of media.

Individuals involved in the New Age movement are likely to review many diverse teachings and practices, especially from Eastern cultures, and formulate their own beliefs based on their experiences, including mystical traditions of most world religions, such as Shamanism, Buddhism and Neopaganism.

Some take the journey on their own, sometimes to explain what they have already experienced. This is the path of the self-initiate, which could mean anything from regarding mysticism as an understanding to awakening, the art of spiritual life, or as a quest for something greater, such as immortality.

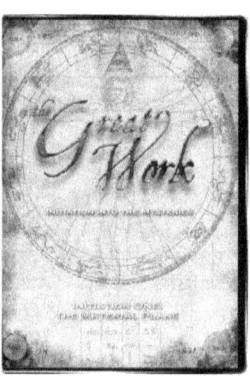

"The Great Work" features a host of leading wisdom teachers including Lon Milo DuQuette, John Anthony West, John Art Rosengarten, PHD, Dr. John F. Demartini, Georgia Lambert, Michael Greer, Pamela Jaye Smith, and Deepak & Roopa Chari.

Created by Chance Gardner, maker of the "Magical Egypt" 9 episode series.

https://www.youtube.com/results?search_query=The+Great+Work+-+Featuring+Lon+MIlo+DuQuette

This series is an excellent teaching of the mystical schools and their ways that extends beyond pure reason and the physical sciences, including the symbolism and unity of many esoteric traditions, with a large emphasis on Masonic and Freemason ways.

Initiation One – The Material Plane

The four elements symbolize the physical, mental, emotional and spiritual bodies, the four states of matter, which are also the basis for the four personality types or quadrants from modern psychology. In the Qaballah, the four holy letters "Yod" "He" "Vav" "He" represent these same four worlds and four parts of the soul. The four suits of the tarot also have this same symbolic meaning. The element of Earth symbolizes the material plane; our bodies and our material life. The initiate's journey begins with an understanding of how we live, act and are influenced by forces on each of the four planes with tested techniques for perfecting and mastering this fundamental aspect of our lives.

Initiation Two - The Mental Plane

The element of Air symbolizes the plane of the mind. The realm of Air signifies lower mind, as opposed to the higher mind which is symbolized by the Fire element. Lower mind is the domain of logic and reason, but it is not the higher aspect of the psyche that we experience as creativity and inspiration. Lower mind can be thought of as a lens that can be trained on whatever we want to manifest in our lives. It can be focused on the good, the destructive, the noble or the wasteful. The mysteries teach that when it is focused on those highest aspects of us and the universe, it is playing its part in the Great Work.

Initiation Three - The Emotional Plane

The element of Water symbolizes the emotional plane. Our blood, our circulatory, our lymphatic systems and our hormones regulate our moods and emotions. Water symbolizes that part of the four-fold psyche that includes emotions, sub-conscious mind, and at the higher end of the spectrum, the phenomenon of intuition. Rather than being something that the initiate must suppress or rise above, the emotional plane must be purified and aligned with the other bodies. Mastery of the emotional plane is a necessary step on the initiate's journey, as the emotions are the ingredient that binds the lower two worlds with the higher two. Join our initiators and educators as we explore time-tested formulae for perfecting this aspect of ourselves, and understanding its role in the Great Work.

Initiation Four - The Plane of Will

The element of Fire symbolizes the plane of will. It is known as the higher mind, the subtle body, our higher self, and so on. The mysterious cosmic fire affects us on all four registers, body, mind, emotions, and spirit.

On the material plane, it is the invisible life force that connects and sustains all matter. It is life, light, sustenance through photosynthesis, and the circulation of all frequencies of life through the universe.

On the mental plane, the cosmic fire reveals itself as creativity, imagination, innovation and Gnosis.

On the emotional plane it reveals itself as our passions, our loves, our affinities and the values we most closely resonate with.

On the highest plane, the cosmic fire manifests as our true will. Not to be confused with simple willpower, our true will is our inborn sense of our place, our path and our roll in the Universe.

The Fire initiation reveals methods for discovering nurturing, and giving expression to the inner fire on all the planes of existence.

Initiation Five - The Quintessence

The mysterious fifth element is the force that binds and animates matter, and at the same time, keeps the elements separate from one another. When the fifth element withdraws from a living form, it immediately begins to disintegrate back into its components.

The Quintessence also symbolizes an emergent property, a rare state of consciousness not accessible under normal conditions. One that is the result of an integration of the four bodies (body, mind and emotions aligned under will) and then a synthesis of the integrated mortal self with the higher self, the Universal Mind.

Esotericism on YouTube
https://www.youtube.com/results?search_query=Esotericism

Mysticism on YouTube
https://www.youtube.com/results?search_query=Mysticism

Law of Attraction on Steroids

An awakening with the Law of Attraction often results in immediate manifestations. It's almost as if we share a primal sub-consciousness that is community oriented. If we need to learn a lesson, wonder how something could possibly work the way it does, want a new better paying job, or you just want more casual encounters with the opposite sex, opportunities will present themselves like never before.

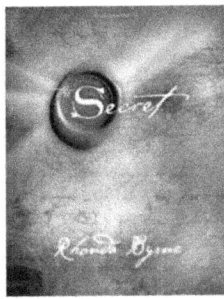

The Secret is a best-selling book and DVD written by Rhonda Byme. It is based on the universe being governed by a natural law called the law of attraction, which is said to work by attracting into a person's life the experiences, situations, events that "match the frequency" which match the person's thought and feelings. Therefore, it claims that positive thinking can create life-changing results, such as health, wealth and happiness.

"Thoughts are magnetic, and thoughts have a frequency" the book assures us. "As you think, those thoughts are sent out into the universe and they magnetically attract all like things that are on the same frequency. Everything sent out returns to the source. And that source is you." It is said that as we think and feel, this natural law of "Like attracts like" is sent out into the universe which attracts back to us events and circumstances on the same frequency, which is another spin on the "Mind Over Matter" philosophy.

The Secret First 20 Minutes
https://www.youtube.com/results?search_query=The+Secret+First+20+Minutes

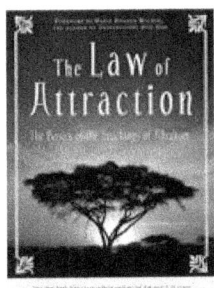

Abraham-Hicks has described themselves as "a group consciousness from the non-physical dimension" whose teachings and wisdom is channeled through Esther Hicks, one of the foremost teachers in the field of the Law of Attraction.

Ester herself calls Abraham "infinite intelligence"

Abraham-Hicks Website:
http://www.abraham-hicks.com/

Abraham-Hicks on YouTube:
https://www.youtube.com/results?search_query=Abraham-Hicks

A synopsis of Abraham-Hicks teachings are clear and easy to understand as put forth on the Abraham-Hicks website:

147

1. You are a physical extension of that which is non-physical.
2. You are here in the body because you chose to be here.
3. The basis of your life is freedom. The purpose of your life is joy.
4. You are a creator; you create with your every thought.
5. Anything that you can imagine is yours to be or do or have.
6. As you are choosing your thoughts, your emotions are guiding you.
7. The universe adores you for it knows your broadest intentions
8. Relax into your natural well-being. All is well (Really it is!)
9. You are a creator of thought ways on your unique path to joy.
10. Actions to be taken are possessions to be exchanges are by products of your focus on joy.
11. You may appropriately depart your body without illness or pain.
12. You can nit die; you are everlasting life.

Advanced Concentration Meditation

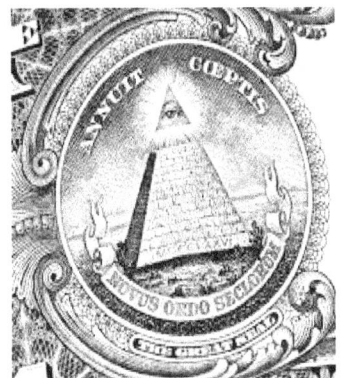 On the back of the dollar bill is a Freemason symbol. Just look at all the symbolism in Washington D.C. to recognize that it is Masonic. The Hollywood interpretation of this symbol would have us believe it's the "All Seeing Eye" or "Eye of Horus", which is an ancient Egyptian symbol of "protection and royal power". Since the eye itself does not look Egyptian, even though it is with a pyramid, the other interpretation would be the "Eye of God, looking over the affairs of man in a country continuing to grow".

Perhaps both interpretations are correct, giving this symbol a duel meaning.

Another term that has multiple meanings is "Ascension", in the sense that something of a lower vibration is raised up and becomes a higher vibration. It's referred to as the expansion of awareness, being one with the creator and all of creation. It's the evolution of human consciousness itself. It's the art of shifting from one dimension, plain of existence, vibrational frequency, or consciousness to a higher state. It represents ever higher awakenings.

Hollywood would have us believe that Ascension is the ability to raise ones very matter to pure energy, as portrayed in the Star Wars movie "A New Hope" and the Star Gate series.

Or is this more esoteric knowledge hidden in plain sight?

In mystic traditions, ascension has the meaning of eternal life and immortality, which is portrayed in movies as if it were fiction, hidden in plain sight.

In the Lucy film, staring Scarlett Johansson, and again in the Transcendence film, starring Johnny Depp, ascension has evolved to new highs as the art of becoming a part of everything.

Here we are going to explore all of the above and something more, with Concentration Mediation. This is often considered the hardest form of meditation. It's not easy to find these on the internet either, after all who wants to buy something that makes them work. At the very least, you need to make it fun for everybody, like lumosity.com does.

Step 1 – The Neural Interface

This is a Concentration Meditation and exercise that I came up with and am willing to share. We start by adapting the symbolism of the dollar bill and using it as a neural interface. What did you expect, a keyboard?

This interface has everything needed to promote personal growth and ever higher awakenings. Just substitute "Dan" for your first name, make it your own, and practice with it until you reach a point where it all becomes natural and the interface is no longer needed.

Take a moment to visualize this interface in your mind and continue to do so from time to time until it becomes natural.

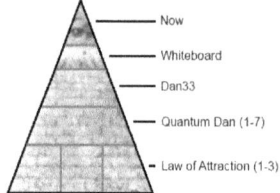

The **"Now"** slot represents living in the moment. Anytime you're having trouble living in the Now, visually reach out and touch the top of the pyramid. Anytime you want to experience something in the Now, like the Law of Attraction, place the energy of those thoughts and feelings in the **"Eye of Now"**.

As an exercise to get started, listen to Beta brainwave entrainments and take those that resonate with you and visually place them and those feelings in the Eye of Now.

The **"Whiteboard"** slot is actually a concept and place that I came up with many years ago. I decided to make it apart of this interface so I could use visual cues to go there.

It is the ultimate expression of inspiration and creative freedom, where lucid dreaming takes place, where day dreaming takes place, where complete and total relaxation takes place, all without any physiological responses or emotional baggage.

There are no deadlines, there is no stress, time has no meaning, and there is no such thing as cost overruns. It serves as a place you can go to be calm and collective under any circumstance. It acts as a buffer, to allow you to decide on a situation before taking it into the Now with any physiological responses that goes with it. It acts as a filter, to allow you to review your creation before committing energy to it, or simply discard the entire model and start anew, like erasing a whiteboard.

I'd like to tell you exactly how I created this wonderful place to visit, but I'm not entirely sure. There was certainly a lot of meditation involved. You can start by listing to Alpha, Theta and Gama brainwave entrainments and place the ones that resonate with you in the Whiteboard.

I'm a computer science major, so the **"Dan33'** slot is the evolution of a life time's worth of work involving the hacking of the human experience. If only we came with an instruction manual, everything would be so much easier.

How it works is outlined in Step 2 through Step 6 below.

Anytime you have a physiological change that you would like to make, like overcoming a health problem or something to do with personal growth, you simply visually put that energy and those feelings in this slot. Here is a short list of some of mine:

- "Reset my Internal Clock to Age 33" – The lifespan of our species should be at least 150 years and there is no reason we should need to succumb to the degenerate disease we call aging. It's certainly not anything I signed on for.
- "Stress Free Lifestyle and Attitude" – Less health problems, quicker healing.
- "More Adaptive Immune and Healing" – Don't participate in the arms race against pathogens when you can win it.
- "Ever Increasing Metabolism, Energy Capacities, Awakenings and Ranges of Vibrational Frequencies"
- "Ever Increasing Access to the Cosmic Consciousness"
- "Repel Energy Spiders and Energy Vampires of All Kinds"

"Quantum Dan (1-7)" is merely a list of abilities you would like to develop along with a scheme for prioritizing them. The idea is to start developing neuro pathways for the ones you want the soonest, by coming up with exercises to develop those skills.

For example, telekinetic abilities are in my #1 slot, so an exercise I often find myself doing is to move my index finger up and down, then try to do it with my focus. You should notice the energy of your focus on your finger, so you will soon realize what really needs to happen is your focus needs to be stronger. My slot #7 is lifting matter to energy, eternal life and immortality.

"**Law of Attraction (1-3)**" is a place where you can take fantasies, desires and dreams from your Whiteboard and store them until you are ready to refine them or bring them into the Now. You can have as many slots as you would like here. I eventually expanded it to 3 sections, through lucid dreaming I came up with 3 sagas, each spanning up to the next 50 years, each with up to 7 full length episodes of things I would like to experience as potential realities.

I can take any part of any of these story lines, like this guide for example, bring it into the Now, with all the inspiration, enthusiasm and motivation that I experienced as it was first conceived. I'd like to tell you the plots to these sages, but one of them in particular could easy be the next Hollywood blockbuster that rivals many of the best ever made, with nothing like you have never seen before, so that's a door I wouldn't mind keeping open.

Step 2 – Cognitive Foundation for Personal Growth

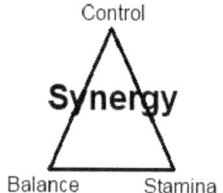

Take a triangle and come up with the three most significant things to you that are necessary to support your endeavors of personal growth. For mine, I used "Control", "Balance" and "Stamina". Now give your triangle a name something like "Personal Growth", "Homeostasis", or "Synergy".

Once you have finished, visually place this triangle on each side of your pyramid interface, signifying the combined effort is greater than the sum of the effects.

Step 3 – Cognitive Progression for Personal Growth

Now take the three points of your root triangle and create three new triangles, each with three points to expand and grow new neuro pathways to your interface. For "Control" you might go with "Power", for "Balance" you might go with "Stability" and "Stamina" you might go with "Endurance" as one of your points on each triangle. There is no right answer here; it just depends on what resonates with you.

Power

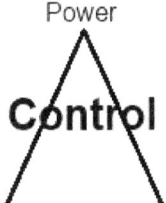

Control

Stability

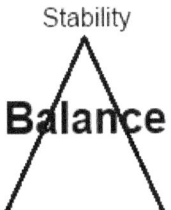

Balance

Endurance

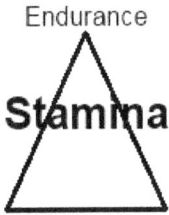

Stamina

Step 4 – Cognitive Evolution for Personal Growth

Now take the nine points of the above triangles and create nine new triangles, each with three points to integrate these neuro pathways to your interface. Take this as many progressions deep as you can, moving up to twenty seven triangles next.

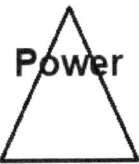

Power

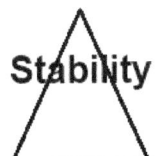

Stability

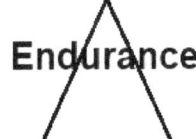

Endurance

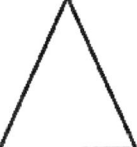

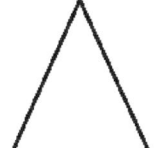

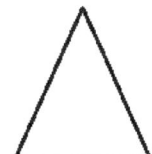

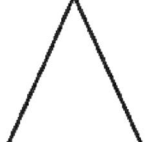

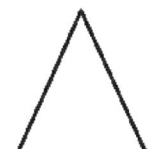

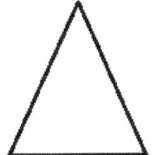

Step 5 – Integration Meditation for Personal Growth

You might be wondering where all this energy that you are placing in your pyramid is actually going? Is it somehow connected to the subconscious mind? The answer is a lot simpler than you think, but you will need to think in the terms of a pseudo "5th Dimension" (duality), find a comfortable place to meditate, and prepare to connect your interface to the very fiber of your being.

Visualize the bottom of your pyramid is a conduit, acting as an amplifier to the energy and frequencies you place in your pyramid. Now imagine that conduit folds space, connecting directly to each of the trillions of trillions of cells and strands of DNA running through your entire mind and body and connecting directly to the 86 billion neurons running through your brain. That may be a reach for some people, so also visually connect it to your heart and heart chakra and let them continuously vibrate your vibrations to your very essence.

Here's where the meditation comes in. Practice placing energy of all kinds in your pyramid; including epiphanies, inspirations, thoughts, ideas, beliefs, desires, and feelings. The more it resonates with you the better. Now practice amplifying those energies and frequencies throughout your heart and to every fiber of your being. This will take more than one session of meditation, but before long it will be very natural and immediate as you work with your interface.

Step 6 – DNA Visualization Meditation for Personal Growth

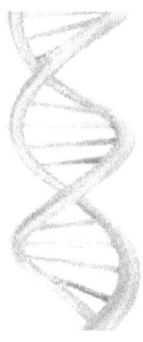

Now imagine each strand of DNA is arranged in a spiral called a double helix. These strands actually split apart during cell division. Each strand has enormous storage capacity and represents your default firmware settings, which is over 99% the same between humans with about 98% of the DNA having unknown functionality even today.

This firmware cannot be directly changed, but it does have the capacity to store tremendous amounts of data and energy, which can be directed.

Now imagine this matrix is capable of resonating a triple helix, a third strand that is pure energy, which is the software operating system to your hardware.

It's really not important to understand how all of the sacred geometry, fractals and mechanics function, but it is important for you to understand that it is within your ability to make basic physiological and personality changes in your life, from

154

better health, better metabolism, better control of weight, increase of your intelligence, improved memory, and even the ability to suppress genes to reduce stress or even become less shy, etc.

All it takes is regular mind-body exercise and practice with this interface, to identify those things that are really important to you and make proactive changes in a way that puts your desires on autopilot.

Hurricane Road Trip

With the last hurricane that came through this area, instead of throwing the usual hurricane party, I turned it into a road trip, chasing the storm back out to sea.

The energy from the storm was flowing through me and my subtle body was highly energetic. It was like reaching new heights on so many levels.

Before getting off the side streets, a bolt of lightning struck a large branch, causing it to become inflamed and fall to the ground. I quickly reacted by putting out the fire using my mind, and it went out before hitting the ground. I turned around to make sure.

As I was driving around a bend in the road, in a foot of water, going much faster than I should have been going, a cop car was coming the other way also moving faster than he should have been. We passed each other at about 2 inches apart. The strange thing is I could see right through my car and felt as if I could hold his car away.

After all the water, my care was running terrible. I energized the engine, and suddenly it started running like a race car.

On the main road, I soured past a gas station, where a cop car turned on his lights and pulled out to come after me. I zapped his car, not only did it stall, he lost all power and his lights went out.

Once I got to the highway, I started manifesting artifacts. Finally, I made hundreds of bubbles with my vision of heaven in them and started passing them out. When I got to the coast, there were many people out and about, some just checking their boats, others walking around, some had to be feeling the sheer energy of the storm.

On the way back, my breaks failed. I stopped for breakfast while waiting to see if I could get the car checked out, but finally gave up and continued with my journey. In time I realized it wasn't going to be a problem, I could make the car stop and it did every time. I never once needed to use the emergency break. Later, my mechanic said it was the worst breaks he had ever seen in his life.

As I approached home, I started manifesting something new, a prototype of a Shakti Quantum Neuron. It would take billions of these to see if it actually worked, but that is something that would have to keep for another day, or perhaps another hurricane.

This could all have been my imagination and synchronicity gone wild, but one thing is for sure, a road trip, or better yet, storm chasing, can be an exhilarating way to get yourself some "me" time.

Neural-Programming

Neural-Programming involves the use of new technologies to reprogram the human brain to help you reach maximum potential.

Your perception of reality is constantly changing with each new experience and each new person who touches your life.

It is often driven by inspiration which isn't always necessary a conscious decision or drive, but yes you do have a lot of influence over it, especially based on what you tune into.

Most of us were raised by our parents and family, was greatly influenced by friends, went to school being programmed by a curriculum, watched TV and radio that was called programming, went to collage with yet another curriculum, used the internet, read books and magazines with yet more bias opinions, was trained on the job by co-workers, and took instruction from at least one boss.

You were born with a body that has most of your physiology and personality defined as a preset of default settings, without a clue about how to change the settings.

When it comes right down to it, just how much of all this programming was really done by you and just how much control or freedom do you think you have over your life, or should I say your perception of your life and reality?

Many of the tools in this guide provide the opportunity for you to learn how to do your own programming, or more so, re-programming of the human experience.

Neuro-Programming Software

Mind WorkStation is an all-in-one toolset for brainwave entrainment that handles the entire process of creating professional entrainment sessions, used on most professionally sold CD's and MP3's. It offers a wide range of audio and visual effects, cutting-edge neural stimulation methods, and easy integration with biofeedback and EEG devices. It features include:

- **Advanced Brainwave Stimulation** - The process of neural stimulation has been perfected and extended in Mind WorkStation. All forms of audio/visual stimulation are possible, along with revolutionary new methods. Everything from Isochronic tones and binaural beats, to sound filtering, AudioStrobe, and on-screen visualizations. Complex filtering methods allow you to use any audio source as the carrier for brainwave entrainment. And, with the new frequency band selector features, it can do this without distorting music.
- **EEG-Driven Stimulation / Biofeedback Integration** - Mind WorkStation is compatible with many popular biofeedback devices and software packages. You can link up to these devices and use them to control entrainment frequencies, to graph their data along with a session, or even to control on-screen visualizations as a form of biofeedback game.
- **Advanced Content** - Mind WorkStation incorporates some exciting new content types, such as the Ambience Generator, which arranges thousands of small audio samples to produce an original ambient environment, such as a forest, a beach, crystal bowls or wind chimes. The best part about this type of content is that it is different every time you use it! Playlists, tone chords, on-screen visualizations and many other unique content types are supported.
- **Intuitive Work Environment** - While Mind WorkStation is easily the most powerful application ever developed for brainwave entrainment, the intuitive interface makes it very simple to perform a variety of common tasks. In fact the

157

program does much of the work for you. The interface is specifically designed for brainwave entrainment and therapy. **Effects -** Mind WorkStation ships with a number of advanced sound effects, including echo, reverb and even "3D sound" features, allowing you to place or move a sound in 3D space. You can adjust the pitch or tempo of any sound file. Filters such as band-pass and low-pass are implemented, along with a wide variety of modulation types such as auto-panning. All of these effects will add to the professionalism of the session and to the psychological effect it has on the client.

Mind WorkStation Website
https://www.transparentcorp.com/products/mindws/

Neuro-Programmer 3 for Windows is the most innovative brainwave entrainment software on the market today and you can try it for free. Here is a list of the most NP3 features:

- 120+ sessions
- AudioStrobe compatible
- Sessions of all types included: *Delta*, *Theta*, *Alpha*, *Beta*, *Gamma* and more complex protocols
- Create your own MP3s and Audio CDs
- Hypnosis Scripting Tools
- Microphone Recording & Text-To-Speech
- Binaural Beats, Monaural and Isochronic Tones supported
- Background Sounds, Music & White Noise generation
- Session Editor, with *Undo*, *Copy/Paste*, *Unlimited Voices* and more
- BioOptimization: using biofeedback device input to create more effective sessions
- Extensive documentation
- Meditation, Relaxation, Sleep and other sessions
- Attention, Learning, Memory and performance sessions

Neuro-Programmer 3 Website
https://www.transparentcorp.com/products/np/

Brainwave Studio for Mac is a universal application that suits people who undergo stressful situations, has trouble falling asleep, or want to meditate. Within a broad selection of available sessions every user will be able to achieve a desired state of mind.

- features star 5 categories (relaxation, stress and anxiety, sleep, meditation, mind training)
- features 40 brainwave entrainment sessions for relaxation
- features star 12 calming melodies to choose from
- features 28 soothing background sounds to create your personalized relaxation experience
- features star High quality Retina graphics
- features Mix ambient sounds together with different volume settings to create your personalized relaxation sounds

Brainwave Studio for Mac
http://www.rcs-software.com/brainwave-studio-for-mac/

BrainWave Generator for Windows is a brain wave stimulation that generates tones with binaural beats. Effects of brain stimulation include relaxation, meditation, learning faster, focusing attention, increasing awareness and self-hypnosis. Examples of possible uses include:

- Relaxation and meditation by entraining your brain into desired states Enhancement of learning capabilities (super learning)
- Sleep induction (for treating insomnia or just for falling asleep quicker)
- Focusing attention and enhancing awareness
- Alleviation of headaches and migraines, as well as other pain
- Preparation for stressful situations
- Self-hypnosis and/or subliminal programming

BrainWave Generator for Windows Website
http://www.bwgen.com/

Subliminal Programming Software

BrainBullet Aim, Fire and Achieve is a new performance technology that zaps your mind with powerful commands, helping you achieve almost anything you desire automatically. Use BrainBullet to effortlessly:

- **Learn new skills at lightning speeds** — absorb facts like a cranial sponge, pick-up information at rapid speeds, understand new ideas and concepts faster than ever.

- **Expand your capacity for thought** — juggle ideas at speed, recognize instant solutions to otherwise complex problems, easily conceive new possibilities and enhance your creativity, effortlessly.
- **Develop a "super glue" memory** — recall information at lightning speeds, gain immediate entry to your unlimited memory banks, remember names and faces with ease and accuracy, every time.
- **Ramp your creativity up to the highest notch** — enjoy the power of truly limitless thought, visualize new and exciting business ventures, rapidly digest new ideas, expand your mind and each of your senses and benefit from variety and adventure in your life.

BrainBullet Aim, Fire and Achieve Website
http://www.brainbullet.com/

MindofWinner for Mac and Windows is an easy to use desktop application, which helps you improve your life and achieve any goal you want. Here is a list of features:

- Simple and easy to use
- Helps you to achieve any goal you want
- 440 messages
- 10 main categories:
  - Personal Development
  - Business
  - Health
  - Love and Relationships
  - Money
  - Skills
  - Brain Power
  - Negative Habits
  - Success in Life
  - Overcome Fears
- You can add custom messages and pictures

Mind of a Winner Website
http://www.mindofwinner.com/subliminal-messages/

MindMaster technology is available to Access the Power of Your Mind and Unleash the Power of Your Subconscious Mind. Their categories include:

- Boost Concentration & Memory
- Increase Self Esteem
- Improve Parenting Skills
- Enhance Business Acumen
- Master Emotions

- Amplify Your Creativity
- Even Lose Weight!

MindMaster Website
http://www.mindmaster.tv/

Subliminal Recording System X1 software allows you to make your own subliminal CD's and MP3's in minutes. Complete step by step subliminal recording system. It is simply the most powerful subliminal message audio recording software on the market.

- Our Subliminal Software makes recording subliminal messages easy.
- Step by step instructions to make your own subliminal CD's or MP3's in just minutes.
- Includes Lifetime Membership to our Online Subliminal Audio Center.
- Integrated 8 track SoundScape Creator for Custom Backgrounds.
- Integrated MP3 Encoder for making Subliminal MP3's.
- Integrated Text to Speech Recorder!
- Integrated Audio Editor!
- Integrated CD to Wav Extractor! - See more at:

Subliminal Recording System X1 Website
http://subliminalrecorder.com/

PowerMind Subliminal Software is able to bypass your mental filters with a 6000 year secret that gets revolutionary results. Here are some of the benefits:

- Release limiting programming and beliefs
- Open your mind to new possibilities
- Follow through on your life's goals effortlessly
- Activate the genius "other" of your brain
- Bypass the resistance that makes any goal
- Break down negative patterns installed subconsciously by others.
- Create confidence, and accelerated learning in any task (even with no experience).
- Align thoughts with the underlying frequency of reality… and reality with your thoughts.
- Consistently move forward towards creating your life's purpose.

PowerMind Subliminal Software Website
http://www.powermind-subliminal.com/

iNeed Motivation, Excellence in Life Enrichment, allows you to browse over 400 powerful subliminal CD and MP3 downloads to help you reshape your life and transform you into a better person. The features include:

- Easy to use. (Press Play on iPod or CD player, sit back, relax, and improve!)
- Simple, **cost-effective** method to better and improve yourself.
- **Fast results!** You can start seeing a difference within 1-2 weeks if not sooner.
- Longer lasting results. A Subliminal CD **bypasses the conscious mind** and inflicts changes deep into the subconscious.
- Relaxing, soothing, and pleasant subliminal audio music recordings to listen to

iNeed Motivation WebSite
http://www.ineedmotivation.com/subliminal-cd.htm

Hypnotictapes.com has 1000+ pre-made state of the art hypnosis recording implants for suggestions into your subconscious mind as a post hypnotic suggestion, as you listen to the subliminal, learning or clearing recordings.

Hypnotictapes.com Website
http://www.hypnotictapes.com/

Subliminal MP's offers 200+ powerful subliminal MP3's to change your negative self-beliefs, eliminate any self-limiting thoughts, and free yourself from long held patters of thinking which are holding you back in life. Download 3 subliminal MP3's and eBook free.

Subliminal MP3's Website
http://www.subliminalmp3s.com/

Additional Tools for Your Tool Belt

Free Online Radio and TV Stations

Almine.TV - Powered by Wavestreaming.com – Sound healing and sacred space technology.

Almine.TV   **Website**
http://www.almine.tv

AmbientRadio.org - Deeply Beautiful Chill out Music - A Heavenly World of Sound - sharing free information & music to help you with your health, healing and happiness.

AmbientRadio.org Website
http://AmbientRadio.org

Deep Energy 2.0 – Music for Sleep, Meditation, Relaxation and Massa
http://tunein.com/radio/Deep-Energy-20---Music-for-Sleep-Meditation-Relaxation-Massa-p402042/

GotRadio - New Age Nuance – Angry, Heavenly, Country, Soulful and Spiritual
http://gotradio.com

Live 365 is an online radio station for free mediation music. Featuring music for spiritual pursuits, primarily aimed as background for meditation, the output is also suitable for healing, hypnotherapy and yoga.

Live 365 Website
http://www.live365.com/stations/energycentre

MeditationFM - Music for Meditation, Yoga, dreaming, sleeping, thinking, relaxation feel the good vibrations, lay back and enjoy

MeditationFM Website
http://meditation.fm

Nature Sounds Radio - Birdsong & Woodland Stream - broadcast relaxing nature sounds, smooth music and soothing soundscapes 24/7, so you can tune in, sit back and chill-out at any time.

Nature Sounds Radio Website
http://www.naturesoundsradio.com

Nirvana Radio - Music for Meditation and Relaxation - We find the best vibrations in the world and we put into our stream. We hope that by listening to this music, you will be able to successfully meditate, heal, work or simply rest after a stressful day.

Nirvana Radio Website
http://www.108.pl

ORSRADIO Newage Radio - Experience the peaceful sounds of New Age spirituality live on New Age. There's no better way to chill out and relax, and we're sure our recipe of rest and relaxation will leave you feeling refreshed and rejuvenated after a long day.

ORSRADIO Newage Radio Website
http://www.orsradio.com/new-age-128k

Pandora Calm Meditation
http://www.pandora.com/calm-meditation

Party Vibe Radio – Ambient, Chill out and Relaxation
https://www.partyvibe.com/forums

Trancemission.FM Radio 128K: New Age 2: new experience of meditation and new age music – trance, new age, pure mediation, and easy meditation livestream. Live your dream and don't dream your life. Enjoy the music on Trancemission.FM

Trancemission.FM Website
http://www.trancemission.fm

Relaxation Ambient Meditation Music - We found the best sounds in the world and we give our flow for your well-being. We hope that by listening to this music, you will meditate, relax and simply rest after stressful day. If you find which this music is useful, it will make us so happy. With ourh best wishes, peace and love.

Relaxation Ambient Meditation Music
http://www.internet-webradio.com

Free MP3 Meditation Downloads

AnmolMehta.com – Mastery of Meditation, Yoga and Zen
http://anmolmehta.com/blog/2010/11/24/free-downloadable-meditation-music-for-relaxation/

Dartmouth College Relaxation Downloads

https://www.dartmouth.edu/~healthed/relax/downloads.html

Free Mindfulness Project Guided Exercises
http://www.freemindfulness.org/download

Guided Meditations – Tara Brack
https://www.tarabrach.com/guided-meditations/

Meditation Music Downloads
http://download.meditation.org.au/meditationmusic.asp

UCLA Mindful Awareness Center Free Guided Meditations
http://marc.ucla.edu/body.cfm?id=22

University of Metaphysical Science Free Audio Meditations
http://umsonline.org/FreeMdtnDownloads.htm

Brainwave Entrainment - Mind Power Mp3
http://www.mindpowermp3.com/what-is-brainwave-entrainment.html

Free Binaural Beats - Free High Quality Binaural Beats!
http://www.free-binaural-beats.com/

Free mp3 downloads – LucidQuest
http://lucidquest.com/music/samples.htm

Binaural beats - Raising My Vibrations
http://www.raisingmyvibrations.com/binaural-beats.html

Free Mp3 Free Music
http://www.findsmarter.com/web?ts=go&q=free+mp3+free+music

Free YouTube Downloaders for Your Mix

Applian Technologies has a free **Freecoder 8 Toolbar** which included a YouTube Downloader, Video Recorder, Audio Recorder, Screen Recorder, Converter, Media Player, MP3 Editor, and Video Search.

For more information on Freecoder
http://freecorder.com/fc8/download.php

Applian Technologies also has a premium **Replay Capture Suite** for Windows and the Max that includes all the tools you need to capture and convert video, Music, and Radio for ANY site.

- Capture All Kinds of Streaming Video & Audio.
- Save Streaming Video, Radio Shows, Music, and More.
- Convert Recorded Files to 36 Popular Formats.
- Edit Audio and Video Files Easily.
- Encrypt personal video files on your PC.
- Includes a one-year subscription to the new Replay Radio!
- Free Demo of each individual product

Replay Media Catcher is the ultimate video downloader. It works great for music too. Its rated #1 by Top Ten Reviews.

Replay Video Capture records ANY video directly from your PC screen. If you can see it, you can capture it in super-high quality.

Replay Music records songs from ANY site or PC program, and adds song info, art and lyrics automatically. Works like magic.

Replay Radio is the best way to enjoy all your favorite radio shows and stations. Automatically records on a schedule

For More Information on Replay Capture Suite
http://applian.com/windows/

Additional Resources

Brain Entrainment CD's – Huge Selection
http://www.compare99.com/compare.html?q=Brain-Entrainment-Cds&ort=Brain-Entrainment-Cds

Brainwave Meditation - When the brain is presented with rhythm similar to its own brainwave frequencies, it synchronizes its own cycles to that same rhythm. This is called Frequency Following Response. Our specifically crafted MP3 sessions will help you to reach those states and much more.

Brainwave Meditation
http://www.brainwave-meditation.net/

Brain Sync Conscious Evolution - Guided Meditation -Experienced meditator or novice, Brain Sync meditation music and guided imagery takes you deep into meditation quickly and easily. Enter the depths of Theta Meditation with these guided meditation CD's and Mp3s.

Brain Sync Conscious Evolution Website
http://www.brainsync.com/audio-store/personal-development/guided-meditation.html

EquiSync brainwave entrainment offers your nervous system a **super fertile atmosphere**, triggering enormously positive transformations in your body and brain.

EquiSync Website
http://eocinstitute.org/meditation/whole_brain_synchronization

Hemi Sync binaural beat CDs can help you experience enhanced mental, physical, and emotional states.

Hemi Sync Website
http://www.hemi-sync.com/

OmHarmonics is engineered to help you instantly relax and live joyfully with no extra effort. It's like having a magic button that gives you wonderful feelings on demand. Can you visualize the kind of impact this would have on your life?

OmHarmonics Website
http://www.omharmonics.com/

167

Top 50 Best "Stress Busting" Smoothies

Free eBook Give Away

Your Secret Coupon Code and URL is

Coupon Code: **BX62S**

https://www.smashwords.com/books/view/618259

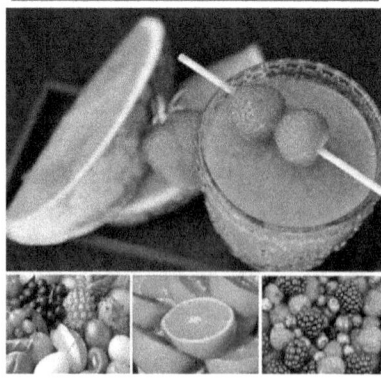

www.ingramcontent.com/pod-product-compliance
Lightning Source LLC
Chambersburg PA
CBHW062207280526
45788CB00001B/476